A FUNERAL FOR MY FAT

A FUNERAL FOR MY FAT

My Journey to Lay One Hundred Pounds to Rest

SHAREE SAMUELS

Skyhorse Publishing

Skyhorse Publishing books may be purchased in bulk at special discounts for sales promotion, corporate gifts, fund-raising, or educational purposes. Special editions can also be created to specifications. For details, contact the Special Sales Department, Skyhorse Publishing, 307 West 36th Street, 11th Floor, New York, NY 10018 or info@skyhorsepublishing.com.

Visit our website at www.skyhorsepublishing.com.

10 9 8 7 6 5 4 3 2 1

Library of Congress Cataloging-in-Publication Data is available on file.

Cover design by Jane Sheppard
Cover photo: iStockphoto

Print ISBN: 978-1-5107-0492-3
Ebook ISBN: 978-1-5107-0493-0

Printed in the United States of America

This book is dedicated to my incredible husband, Andre.

And to my wonderful parents, Brian and Kandyce,
who raised me with love, encouragement,
and a mind-set to accomplish my dreams.
Thank you, Mom and Dad.

Contents

Introduction:
My Best Friend

My best friend and I decided we wanted to lose weight. But working out was too hard for us. We would try, but give up. I thought that running was boring and hurt too much, and I just didn't have the endurance to do traditional gym workouts. My best friend wanted to, though. It was a constant battle between her wanting to work out and me not liking the discomfort I felt. My best friend could keep going; I'd decide that we would stop.

I turned the focus to food.

Before, we would eat junk food whenever we wanted: fast food, cookies, cake, soda, chips, pizza, corn dogs, frozen burritos, pizza pockets. My friend always ate what I ate, even if she really wanted something else.

I was so tired of being overweight! I hated myself for eating copious amounts of junk food. It was her fault! Why didn't she stop me? She knew what my goals were, so why was she not making it easier by helping me stay on track?

We were best friends, but we would fight all the time. It typically ended with me telling her how much I hated her and how ugly and worthless she was. The whole time I was verbally ripping her apart, I knew it was my fault I felt this way. But I was so *frustrated* I had to take it out on her. She didn't stop me from eating the bad food! And she didn't make me work harder. So she was to blame too, the way I saw it.

The next day I decided I was no longer going to eat. *We* were no longer going to eat. She'd complain about how hungry she was. She would constantly ask me when we could eat; I would tell her she was fat. And that she would always be fat if she didn't stop eating. I hated her. I was glad she was hungry. She should be hungry! It was her fault we were both so fat and ugly.

That whole week, all we ate was a cup of soup and an orange.

I felt fat, tired, and ugly. My friend was fat, tired, and ugly.

One night I found myself crying in my bathroom. I just wanted to be pretty! Why could I not be pretty?! I was so ugly. It wasn't fair. My friend was there, so I started telling her how disgusting and ugly she was. I was shouting in her face, screaming that she was a failure and no one would ever want to be with someone as hideous as her. She was fat, and I was fat.

She was exhausted, I could see it in her face. She didn't look healthy, and she looked so sad . . . I stared at her until I couldn't take it anymore. I hit her. And as the mirror broke, I could see my best friend staring back at me through all the broken pieces of the mirror, crying with me.

In this life, we are our own best friend. Friends for life. One body, one life, one team.

How crazy would it be if we talked to our friends that way? If we walked around and constantly told them how unattractive they are, how disgusting their stomach and thighs look? Made comments that no one will love them because of their enormous body? Of course we would never talk to our friends that way; if we did, we wouldn't have many left. If we wouldn't talk to our friends that way . . . why do we feel it's okay to talk to ourselves that way?

When did it become okay to tell yourself how repulsive you are, how you don't deserve to eat because your body is too disgusting to look at? How you're not worthy of happiness because your thighs touch when you walk? It sounds crazy, I know! But, sadly, it happens every day. We are guilty of shattering our "best friend," destroying our own hopes and dreams because of our self-destructive and negative ways. And when did taking up space become the most repulsive thing that a person could do?!

Dark days happen; storm clouds roll in and bring the worst weather with them. So how can you prepare for that?

With rain comes growth. That rain is what makes us stronger and able to complete the climb to our goals. The rain will come with slippery slopes, but that doesn't mean you have to stop and build your life in the muddiest rain puddle you find. You can choose to keep moving forward, even on days when you feel gloomy.

Choosing to love yourself is the most powerful tool you will ever have on your journey. Learning to love yourself is the first step in creating the life you want to live. Your self-love will be a driving force on the days when you feel ready to give up and turn back. When you and your body work as a team and you hold *each other* accountable, you can accomplish anything! When you fuel your body with healthy foods, your body will reward you with endurance to power through those workouts. When you give your body rest days, your body will return the strength to tackle the week. When your body feels good, *you* feel good. When you treat your body poorly, you won't walk around feeling like a rock star. I stopped treating my body like a foreign object working against me, and began to treat my body like the best friend it is. And that friend was the person who helped me reach my goals. I would not be the Sharee I am today without the 256-pound Sharee deciding to fight for our goals.

Sure, self-love sounds easy—I mean, how hard can it be to love yourself? But it is challenging, especially in a society where you're constantly told you need to improve every aspect of your life. From your appearance, the car you drive, and your waist-to-hip ratio, to the technology you use, your job, your relationships, your family, and how you handle stress . . . *nothing* is untouched regarding society's standards of how we can "improve" our lives and become ideal and socially acceptable people. But that doesn't mean you have to conform to societal "norms" or "ideals."

The most valuable and important aspect of any healthy life is your ability to love yourself regardless of your "flaws." And so what if you're flawed?! I actually hate using the term "flaw," because honestly, welcome to real *life,* where thighs touch, or don't touch, and people stare because your legs are stick thin; real *life,* where skin stretches, arms wiggle when you move them, hips have love handles, back fat is a thing, and one boob is bigger than the other. It's not a crime to be a real person. It's not a crime to be thin, and it's not a crime to take up space. It's not a crime to be you. And if someone has a problem with that, it says more about them than you.

But again . . . it's hard. We are talking about self-love here! We are not talking about running a marathon, climbing Mt. Everest, or performing a triple bypass . . . We are talking about self-love! This is no easy task (if you did not read that in a sarcastic voice, please reread with a sarcastic tone). But I know that for some people reading this book right now, self-love does seem impossible. Because self-love exists only in fairy tales with perfectly dressed princesses, and where Prince Charming is always there to save the day. Self-love is found in the fields where the unicorns roam free. Self-love is a concept that seems impossible to achieve, because you are like the person in the opening story. You are the girl or boy constantly fighting with the image in the mirror.

When you look in the mirror and are so enraged and disgusted with what you see, you can't feel anything but hate. You might be big or small; self-love doesn't waltz through the door for those who are skinny, and it doesn't leave the room for those who are big. It doesn't matter what size you are . . . Self-love is a choice and it's not one that is easily made. Self-love takes work, just like any relationship. Except in this relationship, no matter how much you hate, degrade, and despise the other person . . . there is no leaving. You have two options: choose to love yourself and strive to work as a team to accomplish your goals, or choose to hate yourself and spend the entirety of your life struggling with the uphill battle of "I will love myself when I'm perfect."

And just in case you decided that you want to take the challenge of the uphill battle, I'm going to give you some advice: There is no end. There is no medal of "perfection." There is no self-love waiting for you at the top. You will *never* be good enough for yourself if you choose the uphill battle. But you will always be good enough for yourself if you choose to work as a team and strive for the best and healthiest version of yourself. I don't know about you, but I would rather live my life happily than live my life miserably until I'm "perfect." But that could just be me.

So what do you do? How do you overcome the cycle of self-loathing, hate, and destruction? Well, I don't have all the answers. I might be twenty-six years old and oozing with wisdom (haha!), but I don't have all the answers. What I can share is what worked for me and a method that I used on days when hitting the mirror seemed like a "good" choice. What I suggest is, write a letter to yourself; something honest about why you're doing what you're doing, what you're fighting for. And read it on days when you feel, "I don't matter, so why even bother?"

Dear Sharee,

Take a deep breath. Think about how far you have come. Think about the hours of dedication you have put toward your health. Do you really believe you are a failure? So what if the scale didn't show anything this time! It's a stupid lying cow and it will never be on your side! But you know who is on your side? Me.

I am always here for you. I feel your pain, I feel when you're sad, I feel when you're so tired that you want to give up. And it's OKAY to feel that way. It's okay to be tired. Take a rest day. Call your mom. But don't you dare think for one moment that you're useless and haven't accomplished anything! You set out to change your LIFE, not a pair of socks. Life-changing takes time! You knew when you started that it wouldn't happen overnight... But it will happen. I know it will.

Sharee, I am always here for you. I will fight with you, cry with you, and burn some calories with you. But please promise me that you will take care of yourself and me. I can't do this without you. I don't want to lose you and lose us on this journey. This is not about looks (although it will be nice to rock some crop tops someday), this is about the rest of our life: Being healthy. Feeling that sense of belonging and not worrying about our weight.

Buckle up, it's going to be a long journey. But you don't have to do it alone. You have me, God, family, Dre, friends . . . You're not alone. You can do this.

Love yourself,
and love always,
Sharee

Write a letter to yourself; use it as an opportunity to explore what you want to accomplish. What are your goals? What life do you want to create? What encouragement will you need along the way? Write it out. And use it. Use it on those days when a big muddy rain puddle is looking like the place where your life is going to stay. Because, as we begin to walk through my journey, you will see that rain puddles happen more than just once. Throughout this book there will be opportunities for you to reflect on your own life and journey. This book highlights my experiences and my downfalls, and my goal is for my story to spark a movement for you and your journey.

1

A Tour to Rock Bottom

Everyone has a turning point. That moment in their life when they realize they want to change. This moment typically happens when the pain of staying the same is greater than the pain of changing. Sometimes it takes us more than once to see how painful our current state is. For some people, their rock bottom is being humiliated in public by strangers commenting on their weight or food consumption. Other individuals' lowest point is being relentlessly tormented by peers. Some hit their lowest when a significant other leaves them as a result of their weight. Health scares, deteriorating joints, family pressure, spousal "encouragement" . . . Everyone has their turning point. That moment when it's decided that enough is enough. That moment when you're so low, your only option is to go up.

I had a ledge moment in my life. I didn't hit rock bottom until after I fell off the ledge. I thought the ledge was my lowest point, but life has a funny way of making sure you really wake up when you need to. My wake-up call, rock bottom, and teenage-life-shattering moment happened after I started my weight-loss journey. I had already begun the hike up great Mt. Weight Loss, when I became overconfident, stepped too close to the edge, and plummeted to the rocks.

The first day of school was quickly approaching. My senior year of high school. I couldn't believe that in 180 days I would officially be done with high school! One of the best things about a new school year is the new-clothes shopping. Every school year I would go shopping with my mom and get to purchase new clothes, book bags, shoes, and school supplies. My mom and I arrived at the mall and made our way inside. As we shopped at various clothing stores . . . a trend began to develop. Clothing stores that my friends shopped at didn't have my size. I was seventeen years old and a size twenty.

After becoming frustrated with all the stores, my mom saw a store that had some larger-looking women displayed at the front. We went inside and I found a whole store that had clothing in my size—in fact, they didn't carry anything smaller than a twelve. My mom grabbed some jeans for me and I picked a few shirts and went back to the dressing room. I put a pair of jeans and a shirt on and then called my mom to come give her opinion on how I looked.

When my mom walked into the dressing room, I burst into tears. My mom burst into tears too. The whole day was emotionally draining. Store after store, and still nothing would fit. I was seventeen years old and the only place that had jeans large enough was a plus-size clothing store for adult women.

Between the tears I said, "Mom, I don't want to buy old-lady clothes."

And we both sat and cried in the dressing room.

That was my ledge moment, crying in the dressing room with my mom while shopping for my senior-year wardrobe. That moment was not only hard on me, but it was tough for my mom. Her heart broke to see me absolutely crushed and frustrated about my weight. To see her daughter, whom she knew was lovely inside and out, be so emotionally drained, frustrated, and discouraged. A few days later, my mom approached me with the idea of us joining a weight-loss program that met on a weekly basis and had loads of materials to help you be successful.

Before I continue, let me tell you about my mom. She is 5'2½", petite, and thin. She's been a fitness addict for years and even taught fitness classes through all three of her pregnancies. My mom is gorgeous, outgoing, smart, and incredibly fit. My dad is active, handsome, and exceptionally smart. He's a pilot, so we're talking genius IQ levels. Gene pool selection-wise, I was granted top-notch opportunities. This explains my sister—tall, platinum blond hair, ginormous blue eyes, naturally thin. And my brother: tall, tan, handsome, and blessed with the typical teenage-boy metabolism. I was an anomaly even within my own family.

So my mom approached me with the idea of "us" joining this weight-loss program. There was a meeting group not too far from our house. I didn't know much about the program, but I was willing to try anything at this point. My mom wanted to support me, and she had "a stubborn five pounds that she had been trying to lose." So me with my hundred-plus pounds to lose and my mom with her stubborn five pounds walked into our first weight-loss-program meeting.

I was nervous about going. I wasn't sure what to expect. What do people who want to lose weight even talk about? We walked in, found a couple of seats, and sat down. A few people introduced themselves to us and asked how we were doing. Within a few minutes this bright and cheery woman walked to the front and started the meeting.

The meeting began with individuals sharing their weekly accomplishments; some were weight-loss related and others were fitness accomplishments. The atmosphere was full of positivity and support. As more people shared their mini-stories, I looked around the room and saw a thin, petite woman sitting in one of the chairs. She had extremely long hair that reached mid-thigh and was wearing an oversized white T-shirt. She stood out to me because she was so small. I thought to myself, *How could a woman that small possibly need to lose any weight?*

Throughout the meeting, I kept looking over and thinking about why she was attending a weight-loss-program meeting. *She was so small.* When there were ten minutes left in the meeting, the woman leading the gathering shared that a member was receiving a special award today. She explained that the award was the lifetime member achievement award, which is presented to individuals who not only reach their goal weight, but also maintain it for a specific amount of time. Before the name was announced, she shared that this individual had lost over one hundred pounds and was even wearing a shirt to show their "before" picture. She announced the name, and the thin woman with the really long hair walked to the front to collect her award.

My mouth dropped—how could she have lost one hundred pounds?! She was asked to describe how she felt before her weight loss compared to how she felt after. She shared a story I would never forget. It was her turning point, her rock bottom.

One morning she was at a doughnut shop picking up goodies for her co-workers, and while she was walking away, she overheard a group of men say, "Wow, I hope she left some doughnuts for everyone else." And they began mocking her weight. That was her turning point. She went on to lose over one hundred pounds and now wears a shirt with her "before" picture on it.

The meeting ended with me feeling in awe and that I could accomplish the same thing she did. Weight loss didn't seem so daunting after sitting in a room full of people who accomplished it every day. I was excited to join. After the meeting concluded, my mom and I went straight to the grocery store. When we completed our registration for the program we received a bunch of materials to help guide the jump-start weight-loss process. We used the sample grocery list that was provided for our shopping overhaul. We probably had more fun at the grocery store than two people should. But we were so excited. For once I actually felt that I could lose the weight. I could reach my goals. I could look like my mom and my sister. My mom felt it too. I knew she could sense that we had possibly just found the key to my success. We had found the program that was going to help me reach my goals and lose weight. The surge of positive energy fueled our shopping trip. We looked for all the items that were on the list at the grocery store, and we laughed the entire time.

When we got home, we prepackaged all the food and wrote on the outside the servings of each. It seemed so easy. I knew exactly how much I needed to eat every day and all the food was prepared and easily accessible. I just had to grab and go. No more wondering what I needed to eat and feeling guilty for fast-food splurges. I had everything I needed: the food, the materials, the support-group meetings, and my amazing parents. I attended the weekly meetings and the weight slowly began coming off. After two months I had lost eleven pounds. I felt accomplished and proud of myself. I had finally figured out this weight-loss thing. I had the tools, confidence, and attitude to reach my ultimate goal weight. I was down eleven pounds and felt incredible.

Over the next few weeks, my attendance started to decrease, and by month three, I was no longer attending the meetings. I didn't need the meetings anymore; I had lost eleven pounds. Clearly, I had cracked the code of weight loss and was well on my way to prancing around on the beach in an itty-bitty bikini. Weight loss was now a part of me. I understood what I needed to do to reach my goals. It was no longer challenging . . . so I believed that I did not need to put forth the same amount of effort. My body was in weight-loss mode, so I could sit back, relax, and enjoy the weight-loss easy-life process. This whole weight-loss thing, I had mastered it.

I was tiptoeing closer and closer to the ledge, the ledge that was going to send me plummeting to the rocks below. I was creeping closer to my lowest point, and I had no idea. Inflated egos will do that to you, cloud your perception and impair your judgment. Down eleven pounds and I was on top of the world; I could do no wrong. I could reach all my goals and destroy any obstacle that stood in my way. Weight loss was not hard. At least I thought it wasn't.

Eventually, I had to face the consequences of my immaturity. But the extent of my consequnces was yet to be determined. My mom and I sat in the car in silence until I turned to her and said, "Mom . . . I'm nervous. I don't want to see the scale and I don't want to see anybody at this meeting."

"I know, honey," she said, "but this is the first step to getting back on track. I'm nervous too."

I rolled my eyes. *Nervous about what?* I said to myself. *You're small, always have been small, and you lose weight just thinking about losing weight!* The frustration inside me grew. And the anxiety building up inside me was in overdrive. I felt knots in my stomach and wanted to just cry and curl up in a ball away from the world. I wanted to be anywhere else in the world than waiting in the parking lot outside the weight-loss-program building.

I was frustrated with myself. How could I be in this position *again*? Dreading the scale, dreading walking into a meeting, dreading seeing the people who knew I was on a mission to lose weight. I got out of the car, and with my mom a few steps behind me, we walked inside to the program meeting.

I felt like everyone's eyes were on me. Judging me. Asking themselves why I hadn't attended a meeting in so long, when clearly, I had so much weight to lose. Trying to guess how much weight I had gained, in their minds. I kept my head down and tried to avoid eye contact. My face felt red with embarrassment and shame. I hated this feeling. I hated this moment. I wanted to bury my face in humiliation.

It was my turn to weigh in. I took off my jacket and shoes, exhaled, and stepped on the scale. The woman in charge of members' intake wrote down my stats and didn't say anything. She just handed the measurement booklet to me and told us to have a great meeting. My mom and I walked to some empty seats and sat down. I opened up my measurement booklet and tears flooded my eyes. I closed the book and hung my head.

The meeting started, and though I was only a few feet away from the presenter, I felt a thousand miles away from everyone. I stared off in a daze and constantly fought back the tears. I clenched my teeth and took deep breaths in an attempt to stop my tears. My mom put her arm around my shoulders. I don't think she listened to the meeting either. We both sat there and pretended to listen to a meeting about weight loss.

The meeting concluded and we walked out to the car. I didn't have to hide the tears anymore, and I didn't even try. I sobbed. My mom cried too. After a few minutes, I turned to her and said, "Mom, I'm so tired of disappointing myself, you, and Dad! I'm tired of being fat. I'm tired of feeling like a failure! I don't know why I do this to myself! I was doing so good!"

"I know, honey," my mom said. "I know it's hard. What can we do now? What is our next move?" She paused and looked at me.

"I don't know, Mom," I said between tears. "I don't want to give up. I know I can do this because I've shown I can do it before. I'm just so tired of weight loss being so hard. I'm so tired of feeling this way. And I'm tired of having to try so hard for something that seems impossible to commit to. I just don't know how I can do it, Mom."

We didn't conclude the conversation with a game plan or our next goal. I didn't leave the parking lot empowered and ready to take on the world. We drove home with the sound of me crying.

I got home, went upstairs to my room, placed my stats booklet on my dresser, and lay on my bed. I closed my eyes and could still see the most recent entry in my measurement booklet:

Previous weight: 231 . . . Current weight: 256.

We all have those moments. And if you haven't had yours yet, either you're extremely lucky or you're still lingering on the edge. Rock bottom sucks. It blows to be low and feel out of control like an utter failure. Have you reached rock bottom? Are you there right now, trying to decide if you are going to create a game plan or camp there the rest of your life?

Rock bottom doesn't mean defeat and it doesn't define you as a person. But that doesn't make it any less life-altering and heart-crushing. Rock bottom is a wake-up call and the turning point in your life. You will feel defeated and like a failure, but failure is not falling down. Failure is choosing to not stand back up. And if you're reading this book, my guess is that you're not ready to choose failure. You might be struggling to reach your goals, but you're not choosing failure. Failure would be deciding that your health is no longer important. Failure is not accepting that weight loss is hard and will be one of the hardest struggles you endure.

There will be lots of moments on your journey that are filled with hardship. Rock bottom is not the only time when you will have to intentionally choose to be positive. But it is an incredibly powerful moment that can either be used to move forward or allowed to defeat you. To make a rock-bottom moment powerful in a positive way, reflect on it as a teachable moment. Use rock bottom to fuel your passion and desire to move forward. Rock bottom blows—you don't want to be there forever. When you're feeling low on your journey, reflect on where you were before you started the process of weight loss. Reflecting back can help remind you of *why* you eat healthfully and work hard at the gym, so you never feel that low again. So you never have to see that highest number on the scale again. So you never have to feel emotionally, physically, and mentally broken down by your weight.

Unfortunately, I didn't learn from my rock-bottom moment right away. I sat there for a while—I chose to be negative and wallow in self-pity before creating a positive change. So before I ask you to reflect on your rock bottom, I'm going to keep sharing my story . . . because my rock bottom was not over yet.

2

Getting Up

I was at the lowest point in my life and at my highest weight. I let my ego get the best of me and stopped utilizing tools that could help me reach my goals because I thought I knew everything. I ate like a child, I acted like a child, but I was not a child. I was about to turn eighteen years old and I had a serious weight problem.

The sting from my weight-loss program wake-up call remained vivid in my mind. The number 256 lingered and burned in my brain. The defeated feeling of stepping on the scale was replayed over and over in my head. I sulked around for days. While some people are motivated by defeat, and are able to use it as the driving force for a great all-American comeback story, this was not me. I felt like a crushed pile of crap. Once you reach your highest weight, especially when you see that number on a scale, it stays with you. You never forget that moment.

I was sad. Not sad about my weight and my looks because, let's face it, I'd been overweight since I was twelve years old. Being overweight was nothing to be sad about, and it certainly wasn't anything new. I was miserable because I set out to accomplish something and I failed. I created goals that I constantly daydreamed about reaching. I set out to touch the moon . . . and I didn't even leave the earth's atmosphere. I crashed, burned, and drowned in a giant ocean of self-pity. I set out to show my parents that I could be responsible and take charge of my health. The fact is, I couldn't even manage to eat like a grown-up for a few months. I set out to prove people wrong, and I had people whom I wanted to prove wrong, but instead of doing that, I nose-dived and fell right to the ground.

People doubted my willpower. People doubted my abilities. Like the doctor who told me that I would never be small. That I just "wasn't built that way." Because that's a healthy chunk of advice for a fourteen-year-old girl to hear as she manages her way through adolescence and junior high. I wanted to prove wrong the girls who whispered in the hallway that I would be so much prettier if I lost weight. That my face was really pretty, but that I was "kind of big." That was seventh grade.

I wanted to prove wrong the boy who thought it would be funny to give me a bouquet of roses on Valentine's Day. A bouquet of roses that he stole from another girl, who then, in front of a big crowd of their laughing friends, came over and asked for the flowers back. Apparently, a girl like me could receive flowers on Valentine's Day only as a joke. That was eighth grade.

It didn't end in high school either. I was never outright bullied for my weight. No one came up to my face and called me names or threw things at me. But you just know. You know when you're the overweight one. People don't have to tell you what they think about you. You can see it and you can hear the whispers in the hallways, feel the eyes on you whenever you move. I never felt bad about myself or felt that I lacked value and worth. To be honest, I just felt incredibly out of place. I looked older than I was because of my weight. I was in high school and could easily pass as a twenty-five-year-old woman. The weight of the high school athletes was posted along with their bios, and I was heavier than the majority of the male football players. That stung. And unlike them, my 256 pounds were not muscle mass.

A senior in high school, I had hit rock bottom, and I just sat there. I didn't create a game plan. I didn't work hard to revamp my fitness and health. I sat in the pity-puddle I created at the bottom of the rock. I had all the tools I needed. I had two supportive parents who loved me and would give anything to help me achieve my goals. I had a membership to a successful and proven weight-loss company. I had a membership to an all-female gym. I had everything I needed to reach my goals. But instead, I just sat in my pity-puddle and sulked. I pouted because my life was hard as a result of my weight. And losing weight was too hard for me. I couldn't do it.

I sulked about how big of a failure I was. How I would never be able to prove all those people wrong. I would never be able to just walk in a store and grab anything off the rack and be okay. But I wanted that. I wanted that more than anything! To be small. To be fit. To be thin. To be admired for my body. To resemble the girls in movies whom everyone fantasizes about. To be considered the "ideal" beauty. To look like I belonged with my family.

But I wasn't doing anything about it. I had big dreams, big goals, and a big heart. With zero ambition, zero drive, and zero motivation. Over time, I developed a work ethic the size of a fruit fly. I wanted microwave results. I wanted all the effects without the cause. I was my own pitfall. How can you fix that? How do you have a heart-to-heart conversation with yourself? How do you say, "Look, *self*, I've had it. We need a break! You are sabotaging my dreams. Peace out"? Well, it doesn't work that way. You can't ditch yourself. Your only option is to grow and mature into the person who can help you reach your goals. Rock bottom sucks, and the longer you let yourself stay there, the easier it is to set up camp. When you hit the bottom, allow yourself time to pout, cry, and get angry. And *then* get up and get out. Don't do what I did. I sat at rock bottom my entire senior year of high school. I wallowed in self-pity and blamed everything and everyone around me. I whined that life wasn't fair and about why I wasn't born with a body like my sister's.

I was frustrated that my mom was so tiny and I was tall and huge. I cried that my brother could eat anything he wanted and it didn't matter, he stayed thin. All my friends received male attention and had boyfriends, and I was never even asked to one dance in high school. I went to my senior prom with a group of friends who all had their own dates. But rather than do anything positive with my emotions, I let them spiral into more negativity. I allowed everything to be associated with my weight—even though it wasn't. I had irrational beliefs about weight loss and a perfect life. I thought that all my dreams were beyond my reach because of my weight. I allowed myself to believe that everything was related to my weight and that I was unable to control anything that happened to me. It's a vicious cycle that can be easy to stay sucked into. You feel powerless about your weight, so you wallow in self-pity and put yourself down rather than create a plan to help you move forward to your goals.

Rock bottom is a tough place to be. Emotionally, physically, mentally, and spiritually. When you know you're at your lowest point, it can be incredibly difficult to find any sort of motivation to move. The "why bother" feelings set in and you start to feel overwhelmed with pity, doubt, and failure. But just because you feel these things does not mean you *are* these things. You are not a failure because you're overweight. You're not worthless because you don't wear a single-digit clothing size. There are worse things you can be in life than overweight! The amount of space you take up in the world is not a measure of your value as a person. But it's hard to feel positive about yourself when you're emotionally drained and discouraged by your weight. I get it. I've been there.

When you're a hundred pounds overweight, it can be hard for weight loss to seem achievable. One hundred pounds is not something that simply falls off when you make the switch to whole-wheat products. You hear stories all the time about individuals who lost their last stubborn three pounds by cutting out their weeknight ice cream habit. When you're sitting there facing an extra hundred pounds, it's going to take a lot more than cutting out ice cream to drop that much weight. And that's frustrating. You begin to think how cruel the world is—everyone has it so easy compared to you: The person in class who eats fast food every day and still looks like a fitness model. Your co-worker, who constantly brags about their weekend triathlon competitions and appears to flaunt their trim, lean body every day at the office. All while you sit in the staff lounge or a classroom internally crying because your largest-sized pants didn't fit you that morning.

No one understands the unspoken judgment you face on a day-to-day basis. The leers you get while grocery shopping. The shameful glares you get anytime you decide you want some dessert at a restaurant. How you never receive any attention because no one wants to be with someone who looks like you. *Everyone* has it soooo much easier than you! You can't sit down and eat your favorite chips without feeling guilty. Water makes you gag and the thought of drinking it makes you queasy. Soda and juice are the only liquids you're physically able to consume. You can't eat just once piece of cake like everyone else seems to be able to do. Food is constantly on your mind, and it's not the healthy kind. You feel judged everywhere you go. Your weight and size are always on your mind . . . and you feel like your weight and size are always on everyone else's mind too.

It's so tempting to play the victim when it comes to weight. You become bitter toward the world because "people just don't get how hard it is to be overweight." And it's true, being overweight is hard. There is judgment you face on a regular basis. Fat-shaming is a real thing. Body-shaming is a real thing. But does that mean you can't do anything about it? No. This is a huge component to understanding your rock-bottom moment. What are you going to do about it now? What are you going to do with all those negative feelings you have? You have all these negative feelings, emotions, and judgmental experiences that are constantly in your life and on your mind. How can you move on and grow from that? You can't change how people think about you. And I will be honest with you, I am judged just as much now as I was when I was severely overweight. People are rude no matter what size you are. So the moment you stop caring what others think and start focusing on what *you* think, you will be much happier.

Some individuals reading this book might be more than one hundred pounds overweight; you might be 150 pounds overweight. Others might be seventy-five pounds, twenty-five pounds, or fifteen pounds overweight. Losing weight will be hard no matter how much weight you have to lose. And sitting at rock bottom . . . looking up the mountainside of great Mt. Weight Loss . . . that can stop people before they even decide to start. So before you focus on getting up, identify your current placement and life situation. You will not be able to reach the top without accepting that you once were, or currently are, at the bottom.

Reflect on your rock bottom. You need to be able to identify the lows and downfalls in your life if you ever want to get up, get out, and get moving. But know that you *can* get up, get out, and get moving. *Rock bottom is not a permanent place unless you decide you want to stay there.* But know that you don't have to. While it might seem scary to begin the journey of weight loss—it's worth it. And it will get easier as you begin to take the time to learn more about yourself and what you're capable of.

How did you get to rock bottom? If you are right at this moment sitting at your rock bottom, what actions led up to you feeling how you currently feel right now? If you're not at rock bottom, maybe you've already begun to move past your lowest point. How did you feel when you were at your lowest point? Some of you might be on your journey right now, and this book is serving as some extra motivation and inspiration. And others reading this might still be deciding if they even want to start on a journey. It doesn't matter what stage of the journey you're at; everyone can benefit from reflecting on his or her lowest point.

What choices led you to reach rock bottom? I hit my rock bottom because I refused to take responsibility for my actions and continued to eat (and act) like a child. I refused to acknowledge that my weight was a problem. Not everyone will experience significant weight gain as a result of his or her eating habits . . . But I am not that person. What I eat affects me. I gain weight just thinking about unhealthy foods. That's just how God made me. And I can choose to be bitter, or I can choose to acknowledge that my body is highly sensitive to junk food (I break out in pounds) and focus on healthy food instead. You can choose to be bitter about your circumstances or you can choose to grow and learn from them. Either way, the choice is yours to make.

Why is this your rock bottom? What makes your lowest point your lowest point? For me, my rock bottom was a crash of my ego and my highest weight. I saw 256 pounds on the scale. I had gained back the weight I previously lost, plus some more. It was an emotionally overwhelming and crushing experience. An experience that I will never forget. I felt disappointed in myself. I knew all the things I should have been doing to reach my goals, and I was sabotaging myself. That's a hard pill to swallow. I had no one to blame but myself. And I hated it.

Take this time to reflect on your rock bottom. Remember, it's important to identify where you are and where you have been, so you can begin to plan where you want to go.

- Have you hit rock bottom?

  ____

  ____

  ____

- Why is this your rock bottom? What led you to this moment? How long have you been there? Do you plan on moving out or are you going to build camp?

  ____

  ____

  ____

- What is holding you back (i.e., yourself, fear, complacence, family, friends, negative people, time, money, etc.)?

3

Finding Fitness

At 6:30 a.m. on a Saturday, my alarm pierced my beauty slumber. I rolled over and groggily slapped the snooze button. I instantly decided I hated life, and most importantly, hated the personal trainer who scheduled my workout at seven a.m. on a Saturday. I pulled myself out of bed and started to dig through my dresser to find something to wear. I didn't even know how I got myself into this whole personal training special that the new gym was promoting. I should have bowed out when I had to wear a bikini in front of a complete stranger for the "before" picture that came with the promotion.

I didn't own any fancy workout tights or pants; all the cute workout styles never looked good on me anyway. The pants always rolled down if I even thought about moving and the shirts clung to me in all the wrong places. I continued rummaging in my drawers and found some dingy sweatpants and an old camp T-shirt. I pulled the clothes on and glared in the mirror . . . I didn't know what I was expecting to see, but I looked ridiculous. I looked like a girl who had never spent a day at the gym in her entire life. Which was frustrating because I had been attending an all-female gym for a few months, and I still felt like a busted can of biscuits.

I doubt many people will even be there, I told myself. *It's 7:00 a.m. on a Saturday. God isn't even awake yet.*

I sulked down the stairs to the kitchen and sat down at the counter. My stomach felt sick at the thought of eating breakfast. I looked at the clock and saw that I had about ten minutes to get to the gym. I let out a huge sigh, grabbed my car keys, and walked to my car with a giant feeling of dread in my stomach.

I pulled up to the parking lot with a few minutes to spare. I sat in my car and grumbled. I hated mornings. I was tired. I felt fat. And I felt uncomfortable in my own skin and my "gym" clothes. The last thing I wanted to do was work out with someone who looked like she had walked out of a fitness magazine.

I saw my trainer, Jessica, walking around the front desk and figured it was time I make my way inside. Jessica greeted me with a big, perky smile when I opened the door. She asked how I was doing and I laughed and told her that it was 7:00 a.m. on a Saturday, and that I'd been better. She was a morning person. I was (and still am) a noon person.

Jessica was the perfect trainer. She had a great body complemented by fashionable workout clothes. Her arms were toned and lean and I could see her abs through her shirt . . . and it was a loose-fitting shirt! I wanted to look like her. I told myself that was the only positive to working with her. She was constant motivation right in my face. She was like having a walking and talking motivational poster.

Before the workout started, she asked to review my food journal that all the people in the promotion agreed to complete. She scanned through it and then stopped and looked at me. "Why are you eating cookie dough?" she asked.

I was taken aback by her question and instantly went on the defensive and started to argue that the cookie dough was vegan so that meant it was healthy. She shook her head in a mix of amusement and disbelief and shared that no, there is no difference. Cookie dough is cookie dough. And it would not help me reach my goals. I was annoyed.

Who does this girl think she is? I asked myself in my head. *It's vegan!* No animal products were used, so that meant that it was healthy. My whole lifestyle of vegan eating centered on that concept. But Jessica did not agree with my philosophy. Sure, there were also other unhealthy things in my food journal that she found. The next item she asked me about was the potato chips I ate. I could feel myself turning red as she asked me again why I was eating this type of food. I told her that I kept to the portion size and counted out the chips to keep myself "under control." Again it was the wrong answer. She gave me another lecture about how it was all junk and that I couldn't eat it anymore. I hated hearing the word "can't." It instantly made me feel like I was a child. *What do you mean I can't do something?* That's all my brain would think about when she was talking. *I'm eighteen years old—if I'm old enough to vote, I'm old enough to make my own food choices on what I can and* can't *eat!*

You see the mentality I had at that point in my life? I was a child. Age is just a number. You can be twenty-seven years old and still have the eating habits of a seven-year-old, the mentality of "Well, if I want it, I'm going to eat it, because I can." Sure, you can eat whatever you want! You can eat fifteen slices of cake for breakfast if you want! But what you can't control are the consequences of your eating habits. You can't tell your body not to count those extra fifteen hundred calories' worth of potato chips you just consumed. You can't tell your body not to store the fast-food fries you just ate. Yes, you can eat whatever you want! But you can't control what your body decides to do with the foods you eat. You don't get to pick what gets stored as fat and what gets burned for fuel. You have zero say regarding your body's natural process in dealing with calories. That is out of your control. You have control of what you put in your body . . . but not what your body does once you eat it.

That's the point Jessica was trying so hard to make me understand. But I wasn't receptive. I was not ready to accept that with adulthood came responsibility for my health, including my eating habits. I would never reach my goals if I continued to live in denial about the impact that my food choices were having on my life. She wanted me to understand that being vegan was not synonymous with health and weight loss. But I refused to accept that.

She put me on the treadmill to warm up while she went and collected the fitness equipment we would need. To no one's surprise, the gym was empty. I was relieved, because the place was loaded with mirrors . . . and I looked exactly how I felt: out of place and tired. "Ugh, why do gyms need to have so many mirrors?" I groaned to myself. "Do people forget how they look? Why do you want to watch yourself be all sweaty and gross, anyway?"

I hated the gym. I hated the treadmill. I could feel my whole body bouncing around with every step I took and I felt so awkward. Some people seemed to have a natural grace when it came to running. They looked like majestic creatures galloping through fields full of flowers. Not me. I looked like an ogre squeezed into gym clothes, frantically trying to escape the wilderness. While I was on the treadmill the conversation with Jessica replayed over and over in my head.

Who cares if it's cookie dough! It doesn't have any eggs, or dairy. It's basically made from plants! I yelled in my head. *Just because she's a personal trainer doesn't mean she knows everything!* And *she's not even vegan!* My anger continued to grow as my warm-up went on. I knew part of my anger stemmed from the embarrassment of having someone question my eating habits. I was a naturally defensive person, and I knew that. But I still felt justified in some way. Even though I was wrong.

Jessica called me off the treadmill and over to some machine that had lots of weighted cables and benches. She had me start with push-ups with my arms on the bench. She started the countdown at ten. From then on, I wanted to quit. She pushed me through rounds and rounds of all these different types of exercises. Exercises that I had never done before and did *not* enjoy doing. I wanted to pass out.

Somewhere along the third set of moves the room started spinning. I told her that I was going to throw up. And she said, "Sharee, you won't throw up, and if you do, it's okay. Your body is working hard and it's not used to it. But trust me, you can do this."

I hated that workout. I hated that feeling. But I loved Jessica. She taught me that it's okay to be uncomfortable; your body can handle it. It's okay to want to quit . . . but don't. Push through, because discomfort is when change happens. She also taught me to celebrate every victory, even the small ones. Before one of my workout sessions, I was complaining to my mom that I had lost only two pounds. I felt that I was working too hard to lose only two pounds. Well, my mom shared that with Jessica, so Jessica made me complete my entire workout with an extra two pounds on each arm. And two pounds did not feel so small after an hour-long workout!

I stuck with Jessica for eight weeks. I missed some workouts and she was always telling me that I needed to clean up my diet, because even though it's vegan, cookie dough is still cookie dough. I called her the workout Nazi. She was brutal. I didn't walk away from my workouts feeling empowered and addicted to fitness; I actually hated every minute of my workouts with her. But what I did learn was that my body could do more than I thought it could. I was simply holding myself back at the gym and in the kitchen.

I would see Jessica twice a week and was expected to go in on three additional days by myself. I would select times when the gym was half empty because I hated being seen there. When I went on my solo days, I just went through the motions of the workouts. I couldn't push myself as hard as when Jessica was there guiding me. I took more breaks and my form suffered. I just felt so lost and annoyed the entire time.

I had a few friends who would join me occasionally and we would do the whole circuit together. That was fun! But I was not consistent enough to keep a workout partner. The gym just wasn't the place for me. And the kitchen continued to be my downfall.

I struggled the whole eight weeks. My eating habits never improved and my workouts dwindled to just the days when I met with Jessica. I think I lost maybe five pounds the entire eight weeks.

Every pound is a victory. Every movement of the scale in the right direction is worth celebrating. All too easily we tear ourselves down and minimize our victories. Jessica taught me to celebrate them! I learned the importance of focusing on the direction the scale is moving in, not the amount it has moved. And that helped me stay focused on the important things.

My mom, however, did really well and won the competition for best transformation. This is the story of my life: my mom is, and always has been, amazing. The "after" picture photoshoot was just as uncomfortable as the "before" picture photoshoot. I had to stand in front of a random stranger in tiny sport shorts and a sports bra. I hated that feeling. And there were no changes between the two pictures. I was just as bitter as ever toward the gym. But I was vegan, so I was healthy . . . right?

Maybe my experience at the gym and with fitness is similar to yours. Or it might be completely different. For those who have had a different experience, this story is for you . . .

It's about a girl named Sarah. Now Sarah, much like the rest of us, wanted to lose weight, be able to rock her dream wardrobe, and just look and feel better overall. Sarah was tired of feeling "blah" and wanted to pursue her dream of rocking a slim fitness body. Before she went to bed she spent a few minutes browsing fitspiration (fitness plus inspiration) blogs and stories online, and she felt pumped to start her own journey to get a "hot body." The stories online fueled her burning passion to lift all the weights, conquer all the miles, and eat all the healthy food. She fell asleep with thoughts of hot yoga and mason-jar overnight-oat recipes running through her mind.

When Sarah woke up the next morning, she felt ready to take on the day and tackle Operation Get a Hot Body. She eagerly walked to her kitchen to see what healthy options she had for the day. Since she had decided just last night that she wanted to get in the best shape of her life, she didn't have the opportunity to make a trip to the grocery store to complete the "Pantry Overhaul Challenge" she had read about the night before. Rummaging through her pantry, she found an old box of oatmeal stuffed in the back. *Perfect,* Sarah thought, *I can just pair this with half an orange and I'll be set for the day!*

Sarah had read online that "fruit makes you fat," so she didn't want to eat too much fruit but still needed to have some because another article stated that fruit is an important part of a healthy person's diet. Sarah sat down at the table with her half cup of plain oatmeal cooked in water and half an orange. She felt so healthy. She was ready to take on the day! While she ate her breakfast she updated her status on social media to "going to the gym today after work #whoisthisgal #ivegotgoalstoreach." Sarah knew that nothing was officially finalized until documented on social media. She also snapped a picture of her breakfast and uploaded it, along with "#breakfastforfitnessfreaks" and "#operationbikinibod."

After breakfast Sarah got ready for work and decided to park farther away from the entrance to get more steps in her day. She had read some good reviews about a fitness wristband and was looking forward to purchasing one for herself. She walked into her office glowing with pride that she didn't cave and purchase her typical blueberry-lemon muffin and double-chocolate-chunk blended mocha with extra whip and chocolate drizzle. Instead she got a plain brewed coffee with low-fat milk. She was tempted to try soy milk but was unsure about the mixed reviews regarding its potential health risks. And she didn't want to chance ruining her first day of healthy eating. At lunchtime, Sarah ate a salad topped with shredded carrots, but no dressing because of the sodium found in dressings, and she paired her salad with some whole-wheat rice cakes. Sarah looked around to see if any of her co-workers had noticed how healthfully she was eating, but everyone was nose-down on their phones catching up on social media gossip. Typically, she would eat a bacon wrap, smothered with sauce and topped with cheese. She was proud of the choice she made for today's lunch!

She decided now would be a great time to read the special edition fitness magazine she had picked up on her way to work. The cover had a gorgeous model with fantastic abs and stated that the model shared her workout secrets inside. Since Sarah was planning on stopping by the gym on her way home, this would give her some ideas! She eagerly flipped through the magazine, marking the pages that had some recipes she thought she could make at home.

During the last few hours of work, Sarah's stomach was growling. She got a smile across her face just thinking about how healthy she was being, how much weight she was going to lose today, and how she couldn't wait to step on the scale tomorrow! She guessed that she could probably lose five pounds this week if she kept the same eating routine. Her stomach continued to growl, but Sarah drank her lemon-infused water and chewed some sugar-free gum to keep her sweet tooth at bay.

After work, she snacked on a handful of raw almonds while driving to the gym. She had joined the gym online during her lunch break. The online reviews for it seemed positive, and it had a decent membership fee. Sarah pulled into the parking lot and took a selfie before she got out of the car, uploading it with "#itsgymtimebaby." Once inside the gym, she looked around and realized she had no idea what she was doing. Since she had gotten sidetracked purchasing her gym membership at lunch, she had forgotten to take detailed notes on the magazine model's workout secrets. So she decided to start on the treadmill because all the people currently using the treadmills looked skinny, and she wanted to be skinny.

Once on the treadmill, Sarah began to increase her speed and soon felt really good about how fast she was going. But then this tall, slender, gorgeous girl got on the treadmill next to her. And not only did she look like a model, but she was also running so fast she probably competed in the Olympics between photo shoots! Sarah turned up the speed on her treadmill and ran until her legs felt like they were going to fall off and her lungs burned.

Sarah hobbled off the treadmill feeling accomplished that she had run ten seconds longer than the model. She looked around at the free weights and saw an open bench to go sit on. She really had no idea what she was doing . . . but she didn't want people to know. So she picked up a couple of dumbbells and nonchalantly looked around the gym to try to copy what other people were doing. She remembered some random arm moves she had seen on an infomercial one time and did a couple sets of those. Eventually, she lost feeling in her arms and decided that it was a good time to stop.

Sarah practically crawled back to her car. When she got home she was *starving*, so she ate some steamed carrots and a couple of plain rice cakes, and drank two cups of green tea. Sarah went to bed sore, hungry, and feeling "healthy."

Now how long do you think Sarah could keep up with that diet and gym routine? She was doing everything she had read in a magazine and following the advice of what other "healthy" people do . . . But what she was doing was not healthy or maintainable, and it was not about her. Although her intentions were positive—she wanted to create a healthy life for herself and was passionate about doing so—her approach was not reflective of her as a person. Positive intentions do not automatically ensure healthy choices or actions. How many of you are guilty of pulling a Sarah? Of copying what other people do to try to be healthy?

Ultimately, a restrictive low-calorie diet and workouts that center on killing yourself at the gym aren't healthy. While you might not be the social media hashtagging type, the point of the story is that Sarah was extreme in her choices. Although she had positive intentions and the heart and motivation to make the right choices, her method was not reflective of her as a person and it was not reflective of what a maintainable approach to health resembles.

What Sarah experienced is an easy trap to fall into. You wake up one day flooded with motivation and excitement to begin your journey. So you start to implement all these grandiose actions and routines into your day without actually stopping to think, *Is this something that I will be able to keep up with?*

I've done it! I can't tell you how many times I have decided that I am going to train for a marathon and started my training schedule with running seven miles a day. Endurance-wise, I can run seven miles without training. I've done it for fund-raisers and that sort of thing. But my body is not conditioned or trained to withstand the high impact of running day in and day out. I need to *train* to be able to run a marathon. I need to be realistic and allow my body to build up the muscles that are needed to withstand the constant pounding of running.

So even I, a seasoned fitness devotee, can have positive intentions that lead to burnout. It happens to the best of us. Although I have slowly come to accept that running will never be a part of my life, I still cling to the idea that maybe, one day, I will wake up and be able to actually put in the dedicated training needed to complete a marathon. This is highly unlikely because I love to sprint too much to focus on pacing myself—but I can dream! It's okay to have those dreams too. But I have to be realistic and accept that running cannot be my sole form of exercise. It's just not for me.

Don't be a Sarah. Don't mimic what other people do simply because it worked for them. This journey to unleash and uncover the inner healthy you is a long one. And if you don't enjoy it, not only will your journey end abruptly, but you will also hate every minute of it. This is your journey. It needs to be about you. Now I'm not saying that every moment will be perfect and that you will radiate rays of sunshine; that's just unrealistic. What I am saying is that if your journey is about you, when those tough times do happen, you will be more likely to succeed. It will be easy for you to come out on top versus coming out trampled and defeated.

So how do you do that? How do you create a journey about you? Well, I already told you about my experience with a personal trainer, and while I loved my trainer in hindsight, at the time this experience was not what my journey needed. It did not ignite a passion for fitness, and I certainly did not feel excited to work out. So what did it for me? Zumba. I attended my first class with my mom a few months after my personal training trial and I was hooked. I would attend multiple classes a day, five to six times a week! It made me not only enjoy working out but also want to go back! And that is what it takes to be successful on your fitness journey—finding the type of exercise that will make you want to go back. It doesn't have to be Zumba, though. For me personally, running is really difficult. But I understand that some people are really weird and actually enjoy it. They are a rare breed!

When I fell in love with Zumba it allowed me to gain enough confidence to try other group fitness classes. And now I'm a full-blown group fitness addict and instructor. But again—it happened over time. Not overnight. I found a form of fitness that made me feel happy about working out. Finding *your* fitness type is so important. When you find something you love to do, it won't feel like work. You won't find yourself constantly making excuses about why you can't go work out. Exercise will become important to you when it's something you enjoy doing.

The summer my mom and I began attending Zumba classes is when fitness became a part of my life. When my university started that fall, I searched on campus for Zumba classes and discovered that the student recreation center provided Zumba classes amongst other group fitness classes. I started to attend Zumba a few days a week . . . But it wasn't enough for me. Over the summer I had developed the habit of attending five to six times a week, sometimes twice a day! So attending only two classes a week was just not enough. But at the time, that was all my university offered. So I started to scope out the other classes. Since this was my first year at this university, and I had transferred in as a junior with my associate degree, I did not have the typical college dorm-life experience. I already had my own apartment that I shared with an older roommate who had a life of her own. I didn't have any friends whom I could ask to attend classes with me.

I could have let that stop me. I could have justified not trying new things because I didn't want to go alone. This is a common fear people have when trying something new. I've been there! But as much as I didn't want to go alone . . . I wanted to try the other classes. I started with the morning cycling classes. Because they were held at an inconvenient time, I figured that these classes would be smaller and less intimidating. Cycling was hard! Who knew those bike seats could cause so much trauma to your butt-bone? While I didn't prefer waking up at 6:30 a.m., what I did learn is that I liked attending a structured workout class where all I was expected to do was show up and put in the work. I did not have to think about what I was going to do, or what muscle groups to work. I just had to follow directions and make an effort.

I found that cycling was an wonderful workout. And I felt fit leaving the class, as though somehow being one of the 6:30 a.m. people made me more fit than those who attended class later in the day. It gave a good boost to my fitness confidence. So I stuck with it for a while, attending the Tuesday and Thursday cycling classes and the Monday and Wednesday evening Zumba classes. I had a good routine going. But I still felt like I could be doing more. There was an instructor whom I had a gym-crush on (gym-crush: a male or female who attends your gym whom you admire from afar and whose fitness level you are motivated by). She was lean, had your typical "I squat" booty, and was energetic. I wanted to look like her, so I started to attend the classes she taught. Now she taught boot camp. And I had never attended a boot camp–style class before. The first class I attended I stood nervously in the back, watched what equipment the other students grabbed, and followed their lead.

I really had no idea what I was doing, but I just grabbed what everyone else had and found a spot in the back corner—although you can't really hide in a group fitness studio because of all the mirrors. The class was filling up with more students and the instructor walked around saying hi and smiling as students came in. I was nervous. I didn't know what to expect. The music started and the class began. It was filled with lots of jumping, step-ups on the bench, weighted squats with body bars, and killer dumbbell sets, and it ended with an eternity of abdominal work on a floor mat. The forty-five-minute class came to an end and I felt surprisingly amazing. I had survived my first boot camp class and had even gotten a high five from the instructor during class! I felt so fit. I walked around with another boost to my fitness confidence after surviving that class. And from that day on, boot camp was officially added to my weekly workout schedule.

Group fitness was my fitness calling. And that is what ignited my passion for fitness. The positive atmosphere, the guided instruction, the guaranteed effective workout . . . I was hooked! I became a group fitness instructor that following year.

My attitude toward fitness evolved from a hatred of gyms to a love of group fitness classes. I found what worked for me. And that is the *key* to a healthy life complete with fitness: find what makes you happy and find a way to sweat while doing it. You can't be healthy and happy if you're pulling a Sarah. Exercise should be maintainable, realistic, and achievable. Are you making your journey about you? Have you developed an exercise routine that reflects your personal likes and dislikes? Have you even started to exercise? Is your focus on food right now and on planning to exercise "eventually"? Well, that "eventually" is right now—your health depends on it. So now is the time to explore fitness possibilities and be honest with yourself.

Find your passion. Find something that will get you excited about working out. Not everyone is a die-hard fitness addict—I get that. But you don't need to be a die-hard to benefit from fitness. Exercise is an important component to any healthy lifestyle. You need a healthy heart and that is achieved through daily activity.

Use this chart to create a list of possible workouts and exercises to try. Also create an honest list of things you can't commit to. Mine would include running. Running and the elliptical—I can't stand either of those. So what are the exercises on your "Not for Me" list, and what are some exercises that could be on your "Willing to Try" list? This will help you focus on *you* and your journey.

Not for Me	**Willing to Try**

- How many days a week are you willing to dedicate to your fitness journey?

- What time of day works best for you?

- What is holding you back from committing to your fitness journey (i.e., lack of motivation, not enough knowledge, trying to be like Sarah, "I don't know what to try first," "I don't have anyone to go with me," etc.)?

- What steps can you take to overcome your challenges and get started?

____

____

____

____

- Is your journey currently about *you*?

____

____

____

____

4

Grocery Store Tantrums

The taxi driver helped me unload all my suitcases. I'm sure he was thrilled to be lugging around suitcases that had "LOVE PINK" written all over the side in obnoxious metallic print. He set my luggage on the sidewalk and told me to have a good day. I stood in the cold, staring up at the stairs to my new apartment building. As I was staring up, a group of girls walked out of the building doors. One of the girls asked, "Are you Flat 5, Room E?"

I smiled and said, "Yep, that's me!" My journey of studying and living in Edinburgh, Scotland, with four of the greatest roommates (Jessica, Kristin, Megan, and Clarrisa) had begun.

After the adrenaline rush of flying halfway across the world, walking around a beautiful city full of history and castles, and being the person with an "accent" had worn off, I was left with the sinking feeling of "What do vegans eat in Scotland?" None of the grocery stores carried the frozen entrées I ate back at home. Even Oreos, which are a vegan staple in the United States, had dairy in them! And the Scottish version of peanut butter was too sweet. It was more like cookie-peanut-paste than peanut butter, which might sound good, but when you're craving the salty, gooey flavor of *real* peanut butter, cookie-peanut-paste . . . doesn't quite do the trick. It tasted flat and overly sweetened.

My bedroom window overlooked a picturesque park and short-range golf course. The park was a giant patch of well-maintained greens surrounded by ornate stone apartment buildings. It looked like something straight out of a storybook. I could even see a castle from my apartment window. Now that is something you don't wake up to every morning! Living near the park made walking more enjoyable. Walking was also something new to me. I had always had a car. Now all I had were my own legs. You just don't walk places in the suburbs. People go on walks, but you don't walk to the grocery store and to run errands. You drive. Unless you live in the downtown section of a major city, you don't do a lot of walking in the United States.

My first couple of weeks in Scotland were so jam-packed with excitement that my appetite wasn't at its usual high. I bought a box of plain cereal and a carton of soy milk from the grocery store and ate that for every meal. But after a week straight of cereal and soy milk, I started to feel a burning desire for other sources of food. I missed regular breakfast food. I missed my favorite breakfast toaster pastry, or a large bowl of marshmallow cereal complete with a glass of chocolate soy milk. My cravings for marshmallow cereal increased as more and more Irish students moved into the building. I could have *killed* for a vegan chocolate chip muffin! Or a peanut-butter-fudge breakfast cookie. I always loaded up on breakfast cookies at home—so delicious! And who wouldn't want to start the day off with a breakfast cookie?

At nighttime, my snack cravings would set in full force, and I found myself yearning for a big bowl of my beloved jalapeño potato chips. I drooled over thoughts of crispy-fried spring rolls with fried rice from my hometown's best Chinese restaurant. I was in food-culture shock. Even my typical coffee order from my cherished international coffee business was different. How could Scotland and all of Europe not use vanilla-flavored soy milk?! It was madness. I missed my vegan frozen-food aisle in America. The aisle that had all the vegan versions of foods I ditched when I kicked animal by-products: waffles, pizza, ice cream, "chicken" potpies, burgers, fried "chicken" fingers, mac-and-cheese, etc. Scotland was making it so challenging to be a vegan and eat healthfully! What was I supposed to eat now?! How could I maintain a healthy vegan diet if I didn't have my frozen-food aisle full of vegan alternatives?!

I stood in the freezer aisle of the grocery store grabbing package after package and quickly scanning the ingredients for the typical egg and dairy no-no's. After reading countless packages, my hope for finding anything vegan was quickly fading.

Ugh! I screamed in my head. *All I want is some real food! Is it that hard to make a burrito without adding cheese?!* My frustration was increasing and so was my hunger for "real" vegan food. I was grocery shopping with my vegetarian roommate, Megan, and I was jealous of all the options she had for food. She could practically eat everything in the whole store. She had so many possibilities and I had zero. Zero vegan alternatives. My only option at that point was starvation. There I was, standing in a large grocery store, and I was going to starve to death.

Megan grabbed a couple items while I stood there glaring at the freezer door. I contemplated if I could handle the social judgment of throwing various freezer items on the floor. I knew it wasn't socially acceptable behavior, but maybe I could justify my actions because I was so hangry (hungry plus angry). What was I supposed to eat? All the frozen entrées were made with dairy and eggs. I was standing in a sizable grocery store, and there was *nothing* I could eat. And the worst part was . . . the store was a mile away from our flat. We left the store and began our walk home. I pouted the whole way. Megan had loads of groceries. I actually helped her carry some. But I didn't have anything. *Must be nice to have food!* I thought to myself. I wasn't mad at Megan, though, I was just jealous. I was tired of walking and I was tired of eating plain cereal and soy milk.

That night I called my parents and my boyfriend Dre, and told them how lonely I felt. I was happy to be abroad, but missed home. I was grumpy and annoyed that I had nothing to eat. And if I saw another box of plain cereal, I swore that I was going to punch someone! My parents gave me reassuring words and reminded me how amazing the opportunity was to study abroad. Dre didn't want to hear any complaints; I had left him for a year, so he lovingly told me to suck it up.

A couple days later when I was going through, yet again, another pout session at the grocery store, I stumbled upon some hummus. I bought the container and a bag of pretzels. That night my entire flat had a religious experience with hummus. It was so good! We were all so blown away by how delicious the hummus was that we started trying it with everything in the kitchen: bread, broccoli, olives, crackers, and anything else that seemed like it would pair well. My relationship with hummus was formed from that night on. It opened my eyes to a whole new world of eating possibilities in Scotland. Hummus was even on the restaurant menus! Restaurant and café menus were loaded with hummus veggie platters, basil-pesto hummus sandwiches and paninis, and hummus veggie burgers—hummus *everything*.

Although I had been vegan for almost two years by the time I moved to Scotland, I was in no way a healthy vegan. I lived on processed food. I was surrounded by varieties of vegetables, fruits, and whole grains, but all I could look for were the packaged, processed foods. I was a junk-food vegan at her finest, until I no longer had access. When I left for my journey at Napier University in Edinburgh, Scotland, I was 220 pounds. When I returned home, I was 188 pounds.

I lost thirty-two pounds simply by walking and not having access to vegan junk food. In terms of exercise, my level of dedicated exercise decreased while in Scotland. I no longer had access to the awesome group fitness classes my previous university offered. I was still passionate about Zumba, though, so before I left for Scotland I took a Zumba certification course on the off chance that I could teach at a gym while abroad. But there was not a formal student recreation center at my new university, and I didn't feel comfortable applying at a large gym. So my roomies and I would do Zumba in our tiny kitchen about once a week. Other forms of fitness would happen occasionally too. Jessica, Megan, and I would jog the Meadows, and we even hiked up the inactive volcano, Arthur's Seat, once. But there was not much activity in my life. I simply walked and was "forced" to eat simple and unprocessed foods. Who knew apples were vegan? Who knew that you could make a whole meal with just vegetables?

Over time, I started making other foods: rice with tofu and veggies, steamed broccoli with a baked potato, whole-wheat toast with homemade vegetable soups. I learned how to make my own food and stopped relying on the frozen-food sections of grocery stores. Jessica was really good at making soups and showed me how to make my own. She was also the first person who introduced me to quinoa. My eyes were opened to a whole new world of food! But don't get me wrong, I was in no way perfect in terms of healthy eating.

The first time my parents sent a care package, it was full of all my favorite foods. My roommates and I ate so many Oreos and jalapeño potato chips that we were sick for a whole week. But what I learned in Scotland was that I didn't *need* the foods I thought I did. I learned I wasn't actually healthy, I was just vegan. And that this was why my weight loss had halted before traveling to Scotland. I thought that simply being vegan made me healthy. I wasn't being honest with myself about my eating habits. I was hiding behind a vegan label that I had added to my life a few years prior. And I had added it because I thought it sounded cool. I didn't adopt a vegan lifestyle for animals, for the environment, or for its health benefits. I decided to go vegan because I thought it would instantly make me skinny, and because it sounded like a cool thing to say. "Sorry, I can't eat that, I'm vegan." *Bam!* Instant cool points. That's what I thought, at least. I was vegan for the label. And for the idea that vegan equals skinny.

In all honesty, my vegan food habits resembled those of a spoiled child. I might have been an adult by age standards, but I was in no way an adult in my eating habits. Changing to a vegan diet didn't stop my addiction to junk food. I still ate chips, fries, burgers, cake, pizza, ice cream, fried foods, cookies, brownies. I just ate the versions that didn't contain dairy or eggs. But they still had all the sugar, and all the fat. And all the junk was still there. Dre and I had terrible eating habits. We would go buy two bags of tortilla chips and a couple cans of refried beans and that was our dinner. I could eat an entire bag of chips in one sitting! I lived on frozen french fries and cheap Chinese takeout. Just because a dish has vegetables in it does not mean it's healthy. But that was my mentality! And I was still going to the gym and working out!

When I met Dre, I was around 230 pounds, down twenty-six pounds from my highest weight. We met at the library at our university. I was waiting for a group of classmates to show up to study for a test, and he was working at a computer desk with a friend. I thought he and his friend were cute, so I smiled. A few minutes later his friend walked up and said, "My friend thinks you're cute and wants you to call him." He handed me a piece of paper with Dre's phone number. And while I thought it was cheesy that Dre didn't introduce himself to me, obviously something worked because we've been together for six years; married for two.

Dre was working on his major in physical education. He wanted to be a P.E. teacher and was naturally athletic. He quickly became my gym partner. We would go to the gym together in the mornings for my 6:30 a.m. cycling class. He would lift weights while I cycled. And then later in the evening, I would go to Zumba class and he would play basketball. I loved having a gym buddy. Even though we didn't prefer the same method of fitness, it was nice to have someone who would meet me early in the morning on those days when I just didn't feel like going to the gym. But although our fitness lifestyle was great . . . we both suffered with unhealthy eating habits. Dre and I love food. And we loved to eat too much food.

Growing up, food was something I always wanted *more* of. My parents offered healthy options as snacks, but when I reached middle school, I began to make my own food choices. I would show up for breakfast at school early in the morning and purchase breakfast pastries, chocolate milk, and frozen burritos. I think I ate that meal every morning in the seventh and eighth grades. My friends and I would all eat the same things as we sat around the table and talked about typical middle school drama. I was *well* aware of my weight in middle school; by the seventh grade I was already way above two hundred pounds, twice the size of a normal seventh-grade female. But I had no concept that food contributed to my weight. My parents encouraged participation in sports and extracurricular activities, but I was never encouraged to "diet."

When I was about eleven, I would ride my bike next to my dad while he jogged around the neighborhood. My mom was always creating fun ways for me to be active and would invite me to go to the gym with her. My mom and I have some pretty funny stories that we still laugh about today, like our first attempt at the kickboxing program, Tae Bo. And then there was that time when I tripped and fell in step class at the gym. In hindsight, my parents' efforts to encourage a healthy lifestyle, especially healthy eating, went to waste because I was, and still am, extremely stubborn.

As I reached the ages of twelve to thirteen, my parents no longer needed to shape their work schedules to be home when my siblings and I got home from school. So I would eat whatever snacks I wanted: cherry hand pies, cookies, chips, and frozen burritos. Things my parents used as treats, I would devour when they were gone. But here is the thing—I *knew* I was overeating. I would hide the food I was eating. My unhealthy relationship with food was formed because I simply loved to overeat. I did not experience a severe trauma, fall into a depression, or suffer some other circumstance that might lead most individuals down the path of food addiction and developing an unhealthy relationship with food. I simply enjoyed eating too much and did not eat the right things.

My eating habits only became worse as my independence grew. When I turned sixteen, I got a job at a restaurant in a retirement home. When my breaks would come, I would pile up a plate with whatever looked good, grab two or three servings of dessert, and make my way to the juice bar. I became a regular at fast-food places while on lunch break from school. Sleepovers with my best friends often resulted in late-night ice cream runs and candy hauls. This behavior continued until I was a senior in high school . . . and over 230 pounds.

I was not faced with how immature my eating habits were until my time in Scotland, when I pouted at the grocery store because my vegan junk-food options were no longer available. Diet culture is pretty much the same thing. You have a favorite version of your food; let's take pizza as an example. Now if you walk down the frozen-food aisle at the grocery store, you can find all your favorite frozen pizza options in "light" or "fat-free" versions. There is a diet and fat-free version of *everything*. And it's good for you, because it's healthy, right? No. Pizza is pizza. Cookies are cookies. Cake is cake. Stuffed cheese bread is still stuffed cheese bread. You get the idea.

Fruits, vegetables, whole wheat, and healthy forms of proteins . . . all of this was *so* foreign to me! If I was going to eat chicken, it would be fried and served with french fries. I thought the only way to eat vegetables was if they were smothered in ranch dressing. Apple pie could count as fruit, right? When I started my weight-loss program, I continued to eat junk food, but I would just count out the portions. I knew how many points a bag of Skittles cost and I knew how many baked cheese crackers I could have while still staying within my points system. I just floated between diet fads and did what seemed cool. My dad loves to go low carb, and that is what works for him, so I remember joining him a few times and simply eating copious amounts of cheese and tuna fish.

One of my best friends, Kari Anne (she's actually my cousin, so she doesn't have a choice of whether to like me or not!), and I decided to be vegetarian for a few months. It made me feel "healthy" to not be eating fried chicken or hamburgers anymore. So even after our challenge had ended, I decided to continue to stay vegetarian. Vegetarians are healthy, right? Not if you were like me! All I ate, 24/7, were loads of cheese slices on crackers, grilled cheese sandwiches and french fries, frozen vegetarian lasagna, cheese pizza, cheese, cheese, bread, and *more cheese*. You get the idea. Cheese was my thing, plus about four glasses of milk a day. I'm sure I'm not the only person who experienced the cheese-aholic vegetarian phase.

It was during this "healthy" vegetarian phase that I stumbled across the book *Skinny Bitch*. This book was a sassy in-your-face guide to becoming vegan. I was hooked. Yeah! I wanted to be skinny! Reading the book gave me the sense that I could accomplish my goal of being thin by becoming vegan. I read the book in one sitting and walked down the stairs to my parents and stated, "Mom and Dad . . . I'm vegan." And then

I grabbed my car keys and went grocery shopping for my own vegan foods.

I'm sure after I left the house my parents assumed that this was another diet phase I had stumbled upon. But they always supported me regardless. And now, seven years later, I can confidently say that my decision to go vegan was the *best* choice I ever made for my health. Obviously, it did not change my junk-food habits overnight, as made evident by my tantrum at a grocery store in Scotland. But it did eventually lead me to develop healthier eating habits, which I will explain later on, so hang tight.

Before I continue, you are going to either agree or disagree with me. But while reading, please keep in mind that I did not have a healthy relationship with food. I had to hide my food consumption. I was 256 pounds when I graduated from high school. I did *not* have a healthy relationship with food. I was slowly digging my grave with a fork.

Moderation was hard for me. It's still hard for me. I can't eat just one of my favorite foods. "One is too many and a thousand is never enough." This phrase is commonly recited by addicts. I was, and still am, a food addict. Moderation and people with food addictions do not mix. I can't have just one! Sure, I have learned to develop healthy eating habits and am no longer controlled by my desires to overeat, *but* that does not mean that food is not a struggle for me. *I will always have the desire to eat more than the typical person.* And it's that understanding, the understanding that your eating habits are not "normal" and that you have a problem, that will help you create the healthy life you so desperately want and deserve to live.

You might be thinking right now, *How can you say that moderation doesn't work? Does that mean I can never eat my favorite foods again? Doesn't that sound like you have an eating disorder if you believe that everything must be healthy all the time?*

First off, moderation is a great tool! And it works for people who never had a problem in the first place. But let me show you why moderation does not work for those (like me) who have unhealthy relationships with food. Let's say I made cookies for a party, and after the party, all the leftover cookies are on my kitchen table. I look at them, and think how delicious they look, but remind myself that I already had a few at the party. So I move on and continue to clean up the post-party house. But those cookies are still there, calling my name. My mind keeps going back to those cookies. So I make my way over and have just one more. Besides, it was my birthday party, so I'm allowed to enjoy myself, right?

The next morning, the leftover cookies are still on the table. I see them in the morning when I'm trying to eat my healthy breakfast. The cookies look delicious, way better than my oatmeal with blueberries . . . so I decide to have one . . . and the cookies have oatmeal in them, so they are practically breakfast cookies too, right?

Well, now I don't want the cookies to go to waste . . . They already sat out all night . . . They will go bad if I leave them out any longer. So I eat the rest of them. And now I'm frustrated that I ate the cookies, so I think to myself that since I already had the cookies today, I might as well eat the rest of the chips and dip, just to get all the bad food out of the house in one day—because I don't want to waste food. And since my day of healthy eating was already ruined with the cookies, I can just start fresh tomorrow. Bring on the chips and dip.

And that is why moderation does not work for a person with an unhealthy relationship with food. If you have an unhealthy relationship with food, you can't simply "modify" your behavior. If I could have modified my food habits, I would not have been 256 pounds. Telling a person with extremely unhealthy eating habits to eat "in moderation" is like telling an alcoholic to simply learn to control their drinking . . . it just doesn't work. You can't control addictions. You overcome them. But that is not through a process of modification or balance. Moderation to a food addict, or to a person with an unhealthy relationship with food, is like putting a Band-Aid on a broken arm. While it's a form of medical treatment, it does not address the severity of the situation. A broken arm is not healed with a Band-Aid. Food addiction and unhealthy relationships with food are not solved with moderation.

So now you might be thinking, *Okay, so if you don't believe that moderation works for everyone, then what do you support?* Hold on, we will get there. Moderation does not work for alcoholics. You can't tell an alcoholic, "This one shot won't affect you." Moderation does not work for drug addicts. You can't tell a drug addict, "This one hit won't affect you; you can just bounce back to being clean afterward." Moderation works for those who never had a problem in the first place. If you have to "modify," you have a problem. If you have to hide your food in fear of judgment, you have a problem. And identifying that problem is the first step to overcoming it. Just like with any unhealthy relationship or addiction.

I had a problem with food. I couldn't control myself around my favorite foods, I just wanted *more* of them. And when I realized that, I stopped blaming myself for a lack of self-control and decided that I would make a game plan so I could be successful. Does that make me a weak person? I don't think so; I developed my strength through planning, not through my ability to have only one piece of cake. I devoted my time and energy to creating a healthy environment around me. I didn't wallow in the fact that I'm a weakling in terms of self-control with food. So what?! People have issues; it's okay to be weak with food. What is not okay is allowing that to continue to hold you back when you *can* find ways to overcome it.

So how did I overcome my lack of food control without using moderation? I stopped buying foods that I couldn't say no to. You will not find chips in my house. There is no ice cream in my freezer. I don't keep a stocked cookie jar. I don't have a candy stash. If I don't buy it . . . I can't eat it. And when I do have treats, it's when I am at a restaurant where the portion is controlled for me. Over time my strength to say no has increased, because as you continue to develop your healthy habits, your unhealthy habits grow weaker. But until you feel that shift in power, it's best to stop your access to the bad foods. Stop buying junk food. Go to the store with a plan and a list (I include a sample grocery list in the back of this book). And if the food is not on your list . . . it does not go in your cart. You're going to feel a lot more successful when the nighttime munchies strike and you are able to reach for a bag of carrots for crunch versus a jar of chocolate spread and cookies.

Be an adult. Take charge of your healthy habits. Of all the things in life you're powerless over, the ability to build up and strengthen your healthy habits is not one of them. You have control of the strength and effort you put toward your healthy eating habits. Develop it. The more you use it . . . the stronger it becomes. The more times you reach for an apple over a bag of chips, the easier it becomes. Feed your healthy side, not your unhealthy food habits.

Calories? What can I eat? When should I eat? Are carbs okay? While this book is not a detailed guide, I will go over my point of view on these topics later on. First, it's important to identify the unhealthy eating habits that are holding you back. That way, when you start to create the eating lifestyle that will work for you, you can make sure you yourself address and acknowledge the behaviors that led you to become overweight in the first place. It is like if a parent did their child's homework every night. Yes, the child might earn a good grade, but when it comes time to test the child's knowledge on the material, and the parent is not there to provide the answers . . . the child will fail.

If I spoon-feed you a diet plan and a list of things that you can and can't eat, what does that teach you about yourself? How do you grow and develop weight management skills if nothing is ever being taught? Following a meal guide is not teaching. That is dieting. And dieting does not lead to healthy, maintainable habits. It leads to rebounds and crash-dieting cycles. You can be a walking encyclopedia of nutrition, but if you don't acknowledge your unhealthy eating habits and focus on replacing them with healthy ones, all the knowledge and wealth of nutritional advice in the world can't help you. You need to learn about yourself and your habits if you want to be able to maintain your weight after you reach the top of Mt. Weight Loss—that is, your goal weight. You will not maintain your goal weight or a healthy weight range if you don't take time to actually learn what healthy looks like and how it applies to you and your life. Your unhealthy eating habits created a weight problem, and simply depriving them for a few months won't make them go away. You have to acknowledge them and replace them with healthy habits.

Food Checklist

What are the unhealthy food habits that are holding you back? Here is a list of common unhealthy eating habits. Check off your pitfalls.

- ☐ I eat out of boredom.
- ☐ I constantly snack.
- ☐ I am a fast-food junkie.
- ☐ I am a candy addict.
- ☐ Soda is the only liquid I consume.
- ☐ I don't follow recommended serving sizes.
- ☐ My food choices resemble those of a teenage boy: pizza pockets, ranch dressing, frozen burritos, french fries, Pop-Tarts, doughnuts, cookies, frozen pizza, and so on.
- ☐ I wait until I'm starving and then eat the entire house.
- ☐ For me, if it's not smothered in ranch dressing, it's not worth eating.
- ☐ I didn't know people drink water when they are thirsty.
- ☐ I believe apple pie counts as fruit (i.e., I don't eat fruit).
- ☐ I'm an emotional eater: I eat when I'm happy, sad, frustrated, stressed, anxious, and angry. If I'm experiencing an emotion, food is there to feel it too.
- ☐ I fail to plan ahead.
- ☐ I figure, "I'll start eating healthy on Monday" . . . and Monday never comes.

5

On a Mission for Motivation

My feet were beginning to ache and my legs were on the verge of collapsing. *Come on, Sharee, you can do this!* I shouted to myself in my head. My jogging pace was so slow I could have walked faster. But if I switched to a walk, I knew I would collapse and there would be no way I could keep going. I gasped for air as the incline of the hill increased. Sweat continued to pour down my face and my clothes were clinging to me in all the wrong places. But I didn't care how ridiculous and out of place I looked. I was going to finish this five-mile run even if it killed me!

Cars zoomed by me at uncomfortably close distances. I was too focused on the placement of my feet to pay attention to the drivers, but I couldn't help but sense eyes on me. I was the idiot jogging outside in the hot sun on a back-country highway with zero shoulder on the road. I could see my cousin, Kari Anne, in the distance. The gap between us was widening but I was not going to let that slow me down. As long as I kept moving . . . I would be okay. *Just don't stop. Just don't stop. Just don't stop,* I chanted over and over in my head. The consuming feeling of "I'm dying" was rushing through every sore vein and muscle in my body. But I refused to let that stop me.

You can do this, Sharee . . . Just . . . don't . . . stop . . . Please don't stop, I pleaded to myself in my head.

My brain continued to be the only part of my body that pushed me to keep going. If it was up to my body . . . I would have stopped miles ago. I was on the homestretch. I knew all I had to do was make it up this final hill and the remainder of the run would be flat and easy. The only thing between the flat pavement and me was a half-mile stretch of a steadily inclining hill. The heat was relentless and the pavement had zero give. Every single step rattled all the way up to my lower back. My shins were aching and my lungs were burning.

Why did I agree to do this?! I shouted to myself. *Kari Anne enjoys running, that's what she does. I enjoy eating and sitting on the couch . . . That's what I do!* But I didn't want to be that person anymore. I wanted to be like Kari Anne. I wanted to go on five-mile runs in the morning "just because." I wanted to look like a runner with a long, lean body and killer legs. I wanted slim arms and a flat stomach. Running seemed so natural for Kari Anne; it didn't even look like she had to try hard. And here I was, *dying* and clenching onto whatever ounce of life I had left to make it up this hill.

I wanted so badly to stop, to stop jogging and just sit down. But part of me kept pushing to just keep moving. One single strand of some fiber in my body wanted to finish that five-mile run without stopping. But I was disappointed in myself. Here I was, pushing myself the hardest I'd ever done, and all I could feel was my aching body and personal defeat. Why had I done this to myself? I was eighteen years old, and I couldn't even keep up with my cousin who was the same age as me? I was eighteen years old and looked like I was twenty-five because I was one hundred pounds overweight. Tears began to form in my eyes. I didn't know if it was because I was so exhausted or because I was upset with myself. Either way, this run was making me incredibly emotional. The peak of the hill was slowly but surely approaching. I started to count my steps to keep myself focused on anything other than stopping.

Eventually, I could see the gravel driveway to my parents' house, and a wave of relief and emotion swept over me. I finished the jog and collapsed on the porch next to Kari Anne. By the time I arrived she had already caught her breath and gone inside for a glass of water. We sat there in silence with just the sound of my gasping for air surrounding us. I hated that feeling. She made it look so easy. I made it look like I had been run over by death, twice. But in the end—I had done it. I had finished my very first five-mile run and had not stopped once.

I didn't feel motivated after that. In fact I was so sore afterward I didn't do anything fitness related for a whole week. But what I did learn that day is that being fit is hard. And that if I was going to start this journey, I'd better be ready to commit to the hard choices. No one had made me overweight. I had made myself overweight. I was the reason I was 256 pounds. No one had forced me to make the food choices I had made. I was not forced to eat large portions. I did that to myself. I made the conscious choice to eat fast food with my friends. So that meant I was the only one who could lose the weight. No one could do that for me either.

You are the reason you are overweight. And you will be the reason you lose weight. Now you might be thinking, *But Sharee, what about medical conditions?* And you are absolutely 100 percent correct, there are individuals who have medical conditions that significantly impact their weight. But does that mean you're helpless to your health condition for the rest of your life? I don't believe it does.

Here is some tough love: you might have a medical condition, but there is no condition that is forcing you to eat unhealthy food. You have control of the foods you put in your body. Too many people are digging their grave with a fork. Yet they prefer to blame things like: healthy food is gross, they don't have time to work out, they don't have enough energy, they're always on the go, their work schedule is too crazy, they can't afford to eat healthy food, no one else around them eats healthfully, their friends would make fun of them, they don't want anyone to know that they're trying to lose weight . . . Do any of those sound familiar?

So what now? You're motivated, pissed off at yourself, the world, and the people who insulted your weight, and angry at the body-shamers (as you should be, because obese, fat, and overweight are not synonyms of ugly, worthless, and insignificant). And you're ready to start this journey to lose weight. Regain your self-confidence. Show the world the "new and improved" you. Reach your goal weight. Crush your fitness aspirations. *All* these things are just waiting for you to get up, get moving, and eat healthfully. Sounds easy, right?

But anyone who has ever tried to lose weight can tell you that it's not easy. And it's not going to happen overnight. My journey took me five years. Sixty months. One thousand eight hundred twenty-five days. However you want to look at it, it took me five freaking years. It didn't happen just because I wanted it to happen. And it won't happen for you just because you decide you want to lose weight. You have to *make* it happen. Remember, you made yourself overweight . . . and *you* will be the reason you lose weight. Either you want to get in the best shape of your life or you don't. There is no middle. You can't halfway want a goal. Either you want it or you don't. Either you want to reach your ultimate goal weight and goal size . . . or you don't.

So what did I do? I committed my life to my goals. I made them important; I made my health a priority and stopped caring what other people thought about me. And what can you do to reach your goals? Well, I don't have all the magic motivational answers. But what I can share is what worked for me, and my journey.

Motivational Tip Number 1: Commit to your goal and stick to it.

When you finally decide to 100 percent commit to your goal, it will help you make the necessary changes to fulfill that commitment. For me, that meant an all-or-nothing approach. I adopted a vegan lifestyle, designed a schedule that included my workouts, and focused on replacing my unhealthy habits with healthy ones. Was it easy? No way. It sucked. But eventually it became routine and the "norm" for my life. Strive to create a new norm for your life. If you do that, you will never have to focus on losing weight. Your weight will take care of itself, because your whole life will ooze with health.

Now all this positivity is overwhelming, and you might be feeling a rushing sense of "*Yeah, let's do this!*" which is awesome. And I want you to feel that rush of excitement. But do not allow that rush of excitement to impact your ability to properly and appropriately plan ahead. Excitement can lead you to sign up for a marathon in two weeks, when you haven't trained for one in the slightest. Excitement can lead you to purchase three workout programs that are nowhere near your fitness abilities. Excitement can blindingly have you sign up for a sixteen-week training program at a local gym that does not match your goals or your personality.

Excitement is fantastic. But you can't let the powerful sense of excitement crowd your judgment. Eventually, your life will be full of health and eagerness, and you will be able to follow through on those spur-of-the-moment decisions that arise. But until that time, you need to work on building the foundation for your health. Build up and develop your fitness abilities, so you can then confidently sign up for any program or event that gets you pumped. It takes time to build your fitness and healthy eating foundation. Be patient and remain dedicated to the process; the results will follow.

When you stay within your abilities, it's easier to stay committed to reaching your goals. It's difficult to stay motivated when you're in so much pain from the workout the day before that you can't even get out of bed. If you're struggling to sit down on the toilet in the morning, no part of you is going to look forward to an afternoon cycling session. While it's normal to feel sore after a good sweat session, the pain should not be debilitating. That's an indicator that you pushed too hard too soon. You should be able to brush your teeth and take a shower without wincing when you lift your arms. Overenthusiastic exercise can lead to both mental and physical fatigue, and burnout. Commit to your goals but make sure your methods to reach them are appropriate for your fitness abilities, you-centered, and healthy. When your plans of commitment are well thought out and strategic, motivation won't need to be punching you in the face every morning in order for you to have a successful, healthy day. When you plan appropriately, motivation will be able to come and go without you feeling like a complete and utter failure, because the way your journey is set up, motivation won't be the driving force. You will be driven by the diligent preparation you engaged in at the start of your journey, where you focused on making it about you, your goals, and your fitness level.

Motivational Tip Number 2: Find something that you love so getting fit will be fun.

Now I will be straightforward with you: I will never love running. I hate it. To this day running sickens me to my very core. But there are a lot of gorgeous and fit people who swear by running. It changed their life and gave them their dream body. But as amazing as running sounds . . . I can't be a runner. I don't have the mental strength to run. So if I had allowed running to be my workout of choice, would I have reached my goals and been successful in my weight loss? No. I would have given up and been living the never-ending vicious cycle of "I need to lose weight. But I hate working out."

So that is why it's so important to find something you love—or can *learn* to love. I already mentioned my loathsome relationship with personal training and how it made me dread the gym, but how I ended up falling in love with Zumba. That's what sparked my love to work out. You need that spark. Because if you hate your workout, you won't last long. Everything else in your life will seem more important than your workout. And you will find yourself creating excuses so you don't have to go. But if you love your workout, you will find yourself craving those endorphins and desiring the feeling you get after your workout. That is how you can be successful—by finding something you love to do. You will *want* to work out if you enjoy it.

The same thing applies to selecting the time of day to complete your workout. I am not a morning person; I hate mornings. So if the only time I allowed myself to work out was in the mornings, I would never have reached my goals. I would have given up after the first few days. I would have said, "Meh, being fit is just not for me. I'm okay with being overweight . . ." Be realistic with yourself! I like to work out in the evenings. So when I started to attend other fitness classes, I would go to the classes in the evenings. There were a few classes that I could handle in the mornings, like cycling, but even to this day I struggle to wake up early to work out. I'm just not built that way, and it's okay! What matters is that you *do* work out. Some people will tell you that the only effective workouts are the ones you complete before the rest of the world is awake. And they will tell you that you will never reach your goals unless you've already completed a marathon before the birds wake up. But I'm living proof that you can work out after eight p.m. and *still* reach your weight-loss goals. *Calories can't tell time, they just pay attention to when you're burning them.* Do the work. That's what matters.

So create a workout schedule that sets you up for success, because if you don't, you will fail. You will feel guilty every time you miss a workout and succumb to the thinking that you are just not built to be fit, it's too hard, and it's not for you. But you can do it. You just need to be realistic about the time of day you schedule your workouts. Remember, if you don't make your journey about you, you will fail. And it won't be because you don't want it. You can want something really, really, *really* badly and still fail because you didn't set yourself up for success. This is your journey. Make it about you. If it's about you, you will find the time, the place, and the method that you enjoy, and you will reach your goals.

If you hate your workout, you're not going to stick with it. I hate the treadmill. I hate the elliptical. Those are two popular pieces of fitness equipment that I despise and that you will *never* see me on. Does that mean I can't lose weight? No. I did lose weight . . . But I didn't do it on a treadmill; I found something that worked for me and I enjoyed it enough to keep going back. So if you dread the treadmill, hate running, or are sickened at the thought of group fitness classes . . . then don't do it! It's okay to not like typical methods of exercise. Just find one you do enjoy. A way to stay committed is to find something worth committing to. There is nothing motivational about a workout that you hate. There is nothing appealing about exercises that make you cringe at the thought of them. Find something that will make you *want* to go back, something that you can look forward to doing. You will make it work if you enjoy it. And if you don't enjoy it . . . you will find an excuse not to do it.

There is no room for excuses when it comes to your health and fitness goals. Remember, either you want it or you don't. Excuses are in the middle, and when you allow yourself to be in the middle, between your goals and disappointment, you will fail. Acknowledge and accept that only you can lose the weight, and that you need to love what you do in order to be successful.

My views of motivation have evolved and changed as I have grown and entered different stages during my weight-loss journey. I was eighteen years old when I started my journey, and I say my journey officially ended (in terms of reaching a healthy weight range and qualifying for skin removal surgery) at the age of twenty-three. That's a big age difference in terms of maturity and different life experiences. When I was eighteen, I was entering community college and not really sure about my life path. By the time I was twenty-three, I was engaged and entering my second year of graduate school.

When I was eighteen my motivation was driven by vanity; I wanted to look good, fit in, and be a bombshell. This prompted me to try all these different fad diets before I ultimately became vegan, which I decided to do because it seemed cool, like a fashion statement. And you know what? If you're in that phase of motivation right now, where you're driven by outside forces and the desire to look better, that is okay! Not all motivation needs to be intrinsic. My desire to look good is sometimes the only thing that gets my butt to the gym. I want to look good naked. I want to look good in a tiny bikini. That is perfectly acceptable motivation. Hang up a dream or goal outfit in your room and stare at it when thoughts of the gym make you want to crawl back into bed. It's okay to be motivated by outside forces.

As I got older, I realized that internal motivation is a powerful force as well: the desire to not only look healthy but also *be* healthy. I realized that I wanted to have a lower resting heart rate, recover faster between workout intervals, jump higher, squat deeper, etc. I wanted to *be* fit, not just look skinny. Identify your motivators and remind yourself of them when you feel like you're too good to exercise. Or when you feel like your dreams and goals are too big, so why bother.

If someone were to ask me what the hardest thing I had to overcome on my journey was, my answer would not be related to the amount of weight I set out to lose. Sure, losing over one hundred pounds is not an easy task, but it was not the hardest thing I had to overcome on my journey. The hardest thing I had to overcome was my underdeveloped work ethic. I had this false sense of entitlement, thinking I could achieve magnificent weight-loss results simply because I wanted to. I had zero ambition and drive to actually put in the work.

My work ethic was that if I *wanted* something badly enough, I should be able to receive it without needing to alter my life choices to achieve it. That might sound ridiculous, and you might be reading that and thinking, *Wow, what a spoiled child.* But am I really the only person who thinks that way about losing weight? No. In fact, a whole industry makes millions of dollars off of people with this exact same mentality. How many diet pill commercials do you see daily where the person sharing their "amazing" story says, "I lost all this weight and didn't have to exercise or change how I ate"? These commercials are centrally focused on how easy losing weight is with use of a certain product and how you won't need to change or alter your life choices in any way to achieve great results. People buy into this! I admit I've done it! I've bought diet pills from companies that promoted how easily the weight would come off by taking their products. Did they work? No. Because weight loss is hard. And anyone who tells you otherwise is either lying or misinformed. But just because weight loss is hard does not mean it's impossible or unbearable.

That is where there is a common breakdown. When people hear the words "hard" or "difficult" they automatically assume these equate to "impossible" or "too difficult to even try."

When did working hard become this mythical creature that only the extremely fortunate are able to capture? Hard work might not be your preferred method of work . . . but in terms of achieving the goal waiting for you at the top of Mt. Weight Loss, it is your only option. Mt. Weight Loss is not for the faint of heart or for individuals who spend their money on diet pills.

Hard work is not synonymous with unenjoyable or miserable. Save your money for healthy food and end-goal clothes. You don't need to spend it on detox teas, weight-loss pills, or any other "get skinny easy" scheme. Just as an FYI, we have organs in our bodies that do the detox for us. God built us with our own detox system. You don't need a fancy tea, or to drink kale smoothies for seventy-two hours until your toilet is tinted green in order to lose weight. Want a quick detox method to help jump-start your weight loss? Stop eating junk and get serious about changing your lifestyle.

Many days you might find a different reason to be motivated. And some days, you might not have any motivation. The thought of doing anything that will contribute to your weight-loss journey may exhaust you on these days. So what happens then? This is when your commitment to your health and your dedication to creating a lifestyle change come into play. On those days, what do you have written on your weekly schedule? What workouts have you scheduled? Remember, this is not about motivation, it's about dedication. If your workouts are scheduled, you must go. You're the boss for this meeting so you need to show up. And why wouldn't you want to go? You scheduled a workout you enjoy, didn't you? It's not the most motivated individuals who make it to the top, it's those who remain dedicated and diligent. Practice skills that will enforce and strengthen your dedication; don't focus on constantly trying to feel motivated.

On days you don't feel motivated, your dedication to yourself, your goals, and your health will be your driving force. On days you feel awesome and energized, that's when your motivation will shine. Both are important, and you will experience both days of extreme motivation and periods of motivational droughts. By developing a plan that will help you remain dedicated during those droughts, you will continue to climb even when you feel like giving up. Like I said before, this is what worked for me and my journey, so my guess is if it helped me lose weight and reach my goals, it might help you too.

What can help you stay dedicated and focused is developing a personal mission statement. A mission statement is a statement that summarizes your aim, goals, and values for your journey. Creating a formalized mission statement can help you stay focused on those days when you just don't feel like doing anything productive or healthy—those days when all the unhealthy foods seem like the only good foods. A mission statement can help on those days when you feel like every step you take forward, you're pushed two steps back. Those days will happen, so here is a plan to help you stay focused on dedication and not the overwhelming sense of "I don't want to do this anymore."

Here are some examples of weight-loss-journey mission statements:

My mission is to create the best version of myself.

On my journey I will focus on developing healthy habits, creating a healthy life I enjoy, and living my life to the fullest.

I aim to create a healthy life I enjoy and a journey I can be proud of.

I want my story to inspire those around me to dream big, and to show that you can be the person you've always wanted to be.

Now what is your personal mission statement?

____

____

____

____

____

6

"F" for Effort

I stepped on the scale, exhaled, and closed my eyes. After a few agonizing seconds I looked down to read the numbers. "Ugh," I groaned. The number 188 glared back at me. The same three numbers for the past four freaking months! I was beginning to believe that I was just destined to weigh 188 pounds for the rest of my life. *I don't get it!* I screamed to myself in my head. *I lost weight so easily when I lived in Scotland and I wasn't even trying! Now here I am back at home, and I haven't lost a pound in over four months! I'm teaching Zumba two days a week and still eating the same things I ate in Scotland. What gives?!* My internal dialogue continued on for some time.

My year abroad in Scotland came to an end before the summer and I moved back home. I stayed with my parents over the summer break, like I always did, and then moved back to my university campus in the fall. I had one more year left for my bachelor's degree and was determined to continue down the weight-loss path. But I was so frustrated! In Scotland it had come naturally. Because I could no longer survive on vegan junk food, I actually had to learn to eat healthy food. And I also had to walk . . . *everywhere.* Walk to work. Walk to school. Walk to the store. Walk for nights out. Everything I wanted to do included walking. And walking everywhere had added up on the calorie-burning scale.

Back home, I once again had access to my Jeep and all my favorite foods. And as a result, weight loss halted. But I was teaching group fitness classes too. While I lived in Scotland I had taught Zumba to my flatmates in our tiny kitchen, and occasionally we would jog the park trails behind our flat. Nothing had been structured, though. Once I was back home, I actually committed to teaching classes two days a week and attending a few other fitness classes here and there. But no weight loss. Not one single ounce. And I was still eating basically the same things: microwaved potatoes, steamed broccoli, asparagus, and whole-wheat toast. To be honest, I ate that meal almost every day while I lived in Scotland. And I had seen results! I whined to my new roommate, Brea, about how annoying it was to go from losing so much weight without even really trying, to actually trying and seeing no results.

Brea and I could relate on multiple levels. She had struggled with her weight her whole life and had eventually undergone gastric bypass surgery. Now fully recovered from her surgery, she was on her journey to reach her goal weight and create lasting healthy habits. Brea was your typical vegan peace-loving hippie. She even majored in primate behavior and worked with the chimpanzees that used sign language at my university. We were, and still are, best friends. She and I would attend workout classes together throughout the week, and I encouraged her to try my Zumba classes. She became a front-row member. Brea was my go-to person when it came to complaining about my weight-loss plateau. She would also make fun of me for the obnoxious amounts of broccoli I would eat and how the whole house would stink of steamed broccoli.

A few more months went by and the scale continued to glare "188" back at me. My frustration increased and my motivation decreased. My workouts diminished from attending a few extra fitness classes a week, to participating only in the two classes that I taught. I was still happy with myself and proud of my weight loss in Scotland, but sad that it appeared that I was at the end of my journey. I didn't have visible abs, my arms looked flabby, and my bully button was hidden by a "frown" of skin. I didn't feel like I had reached the finish line. I felt emotionally deflated.

Although I was nowhere near rock bottom, I couldn't help but feel the same sense of defeat. I was sitting at the halfway mark of the trek up Mt. Weight Loss. I had found a comfortable ledge to rest and make camp—and I didn't even know it. Scotland was the trail that I was able to coast along. It wasn't too steep but still required some effort on my part. And I was able to maintain a steady pace and make some headway. Now I was sitting on the ledge right before the steepest part of the climb, the part that requires you to grit your teeth and put on your big-girl boots and get to work. The part where a hike turns into rock climbing, I was almost there. I just needed to pack up camp first.

Christmas was approaching. I was excited to spend a whole month home with my family and enjoy a much-needed break from school. My mom asked me what I wanted from "Santa" and I wasn't sure. If Santa could bring me a scale that said something other than 188, that would be great! But something was lingering in my mind. Late one night I had seen an infomercial on TV promoting a super-intense workout program. The program was designed to deliver amazing results in sixty days, complete with different daily in-home workouts and an easy-to-follow nutrition guide. That's what I wanted from Santa. And Santa did not disappoint.

Along with the new workout program, I also received some new exercise clothes and fitness accessories. I was so ready and determined to crush my goals! I was determined to break up with 188 once and for all! By this point I had been at 188 pounds for seven months. My family and I sat in the living room talking and admiring all the gifts. My mom asked me when I was going to start my new program. I talked nervously about how the nutrition guide seemed different and how I was excited and nervous at the same time. The guide would require me to get creative on making vegan swaps, but it was doable. My mom and I sat down at the kitchen table and looked through the nutrition guide. We talked about the new recipes we could make and what groceries we would need to buy. My mom seemed more excited than me and went online to purchase the workout program for herself too! We both agreed we would start after New Year's. It would be our resolution to complete the program. My dad sat on the couch rolling his eyes; he knew anytime my mom got excited about something, he would be "encouraged" (in his words, "forced") to be excited about it too.

The program details made the workouts seem so hard-core. I was ready for this challenge! I was ready to release my inner fitness girl . . . if I even had one to release. I wasn't 100 percent sure yet. But what I did know was that I was ready to not weigh 188 pounds and I was ready to keep climbing up Mt. Weight Loss. I was tired of camping and ready to get back on the trail.

New Year's came and went, and within a few days I was back at school. I eagerly told Brea about the new program I had received and encouraged her to do it with me. She wasn't too thrilled but agreed to participate if her schedule allowed. I hung up the workout schedule on my bedroom wall and headed to the grocery store in town to purchase all the food I would need to set myself up for success. Brea and I were such nerds, grocery store runs were a favorite pastime and we'd routinely end up purchasing clothes and other things we absolutely did not need. But that's what happens when the best grocery store in town is also a superstore that stocks everything from lawn mowers to apparel.

I went through all the aisles grabbing all the things I needed, attempting to mentally figure out how many fresh fruits and vegetables I would require for the week. We made our purchases and headed back to our apartment. Brea had to work a night shift, so she wouldn't be joining me for my first workout. But she helped me arrange the living room furniture so I wouldn't give myself a concussion on an end table. She left for work and I laced up my workout shoes and hit play on the DVD player.

After the first few minutes, the initial excitement and adrenaline rush I had gotten from anticipating a new workout program had worn off. I was now facing a workout so challenging I started to feel tears well up in my eyes halfway through the workout. The whole workout was only twenty-five minutes and every minute made me feel exhausted and demoralized. I had thought I was semi-fit! *I taught fitness classes!* I screamed to myself in my head. *I should be able to complete this without feeling like my heart is going to explode!*

The twenty-five minutes felt like an eternity. And once that eternity was over I lay on the living room floor a sweaty, exhausted, and defeated 188-pound blob. I don't know how long I lay there to catch my breath, but eventually I found enough strength to make it to my room and call my mom. "Mom!" I screamed into the phone.

"Honey, what's wrong?!" she stated with concern in her voice.

"I just finished the first workout!" I wailed into the phone. "It was so hard! I thought I was somewhat in shape! I can't believe it was only twenty-five minutes and it was that hard! I don't know how I can do sixty days of this!" My mom agreed with me that it was one of the hardest workouts she had ever done, but encouraged me to just think about how great we would look and feel after sixty days. My mom was always my voice of reason when I felt like giving up. She was always that constant motivator and voice of encouragement at the times when I needed it most. And this was one of those times.

I knew she was right. And I didn't actually want to give up, I was just not expecting the program to be as difficult as it was. But this was just the first workout! And it wasn't even full length! Shortly after talking to my mom, I called Dre and complained about how hard it was. He was excited for me and encouraged me to stick with it. He didn't want to commit to the program but agreed to try one or two workouts with me to see what all the hype was about. Needless to say, when the time came around for him to try one out, he also collapsed from exhaustion. Dre and I were and still are each other's number-one workout buddies, but we enjoy different kinds of fitness. We don't have to complete the same workout in order to be supportive of one another's goals.

I didn't have a scale in my apartment, so the only time to weigh myself was during my bimonthly visits to my parents' house. After sticking with the program for two weeks, I was anxious to see what the scale would read. The first few days into the program I caught the flu and was out for a couple days. I decided I would start the program over again and was nervous that it might have impacted my results. However, I was diligently following the meal plan. I would portion out my meals in the morning and pack my snacks for class. I was always prepared for when hunger would strike! But still, I didn't know what to expect. And the way my body had been the past seven months, it was not in the business of losing weight.

The morning for me to weigh myself came. Two weeks had passed since I had last seen 188—fourteen days of pushing myself with this new program and teaching my fitness classes at school. I started to break into a sweat looking at the scale. I took a deep breath, stepped on the scale, and exhaled. I waited a few seconds before I looked down. When I looked down, I was instantly filled with joy! The scale read 181! I had lost seven pounds—seven pounds in two weeks after not losing a single pound in seven months! I put my clothes on (I do naked weigh-ins; every ounce counts) and ran out to find my mom.

She was overjoyed too! We spent the whole weekend comparing stories on how sore we were and swapping recipes and substitutions from the nutrition guide. It was a good weekend. I had finally found something that my body responded to: dedicated food intake, intense workouts, and consistency. So it wasn't that complicated after all. This may sound like a pretty standard method for weight loss, but in my case, I needed a wake-up call. My body was finished responding to me simply trying to coast my way through weight loss. I was filled with excitement, and nervousness. I had survived the first fourteen days, but the question remained: Would I be able to last the whole sixty? I called Dre and shared my news. He was so proud of me and shared that he would encourage and help me stick with it. He was always so supportive; even if we didn't prefer the same methods of fitness, we always supported each other's goals.

I said farewell to my parents and headed back to school. Brea was ecstatic for me and made jokes that sixty days of not being able to walk straight because of sore muscles is not that long. I shared the news with a few members in my fitness classes, and over time more and more people kept asking about my progress. The workouts never became easier, but I could feel myself becoming stronger and I was able to push myself harder. My clothes started to feel looser and I would get random compliments on how great I was looking. I still experienced slight anxiety at the sight of the scale, but my effort was paying off. The numbers continued to go down.

After about sixty days, I was down to 159 pounds and a size six (I started at a size fourteen). I was the smallest I had ever been in my entire life! I was wearing clothes that I had never been able to comfortably wear before. I looked in the mirror and I felt amazing! I was officially down ninety-seven pounds from my highest weight. I could have given up at 188 pounds. I could have decided that I was done with losing weight after seven months of not losing one single pound. But I didn't. So what changed? My effort. My honesty with myself. My dedication. My comfort level.

I had reached a place of complacency in my journey. When I lived in Scotland my food habits drastically changed due to limited junk-food opportunities, and I was forced to walk everywhere. That shocked my body enough to lose over thirty pounds. But then I came back home and although my eating habits stayed similar, my walking decreased and I did not find enough additional methods of exercise. My body had adjusted and I was left with two options: either work harder or camp out. In the weight-loss realm this is called a "plateau."

Seven months is a long plateau. Some people will experience plateaus for a few weeks, while other people experience situations similar to mine. Now I could have given up, but I didn't. And if you're experiencing a plateau right now, you don't need to give up either. Remember, weight loss is science, not magic. It's about finding the right equation for your body, figuring out what the reason is for your plateau. You don't need to freak out and give up. What you need to do is check your E.F.F.O.R.T. This stands for Exercise, Food, Focus, Organization, Rest, and Time. All of these areas are important, and by exploring them individually you can begin to target the areas of your "equation" that might need revamping or restructuring.

Exercise: In my case, this was a huge component of the reason I was stuck at 188 pounds for so long. My body's equation is 100 percent exercise and 100 percent healthy eating. If I start to stray from either of those or begin dedicating more time to one or the other, I stop seeing results. Not everyone is the same, so that is why it's so important to take the time to evaluate the equation that works best for your body. Also keep in mind that our bodies need change. My seven-month plateau is a perfect example of how our bodies can stop responding to methods that previously worked. Initially, my equation was 100 percent food and about 25 percent exercise. But after thirty pounds of weight loss, my body no longer responded to that equation. I had to switch it up and step it up about a thousand notches, to a whole other level of crazy fitness. *But* . . . it worked!

So evaluate your exercise. Are you pushing yourself enough? Are the workouts a reflection of *you* on your journey? Remember, you don't want to pull a Sarah and try to be someone you're not.

Exercise may be something you have not yet added to your journey. I get it; some people don't like fitness and would rather focus on food. And if that works for you, great! But I will always support living a healthy, active life. That doesn't mean you need to run a marathon every weekend. It can mean scheduling a time in your day when you walk the dog for thirty minutes. But if you don't have a scheduled exercise regimen, and you've stopped seeing weight-loss results, it might be time to reconsider your equation. Our bodies change, and what worked for you before might need to be updated. And that is okay! It means your body is improving. So while I know that plateaus are frustrating, remind yourself that your body is trying to say, "Hey, I'm stronger than this! We *can* do more." While it's annoying . . . it's kind of a confidence booster too. It just depends on how you look at it.

If you're the opposite, and you already have a dedicated workout schedule, it might be time for you to amp up the intensity of your fitness. Your dedication to your fitness has paid off in the sense that now you need to work harder to continue to see results. If you're comfortable with your current workouts you will not see change. Change does not happen in our comfort zone. Change happens when your body is forced to work harder. Losing weight and creating a healthy life take work . . . but it's worth it. So seek out those challenging workouts—the workouts that leave you in a puddle of sweat on the floor, the workouts where you can increase your resistance or challenge different muscle groups. Mix things up. Much like how you would get bored of eating the same meal day after day, our bodies like some variety in terms of exercise. Find something that will challenge you in a whole new way and embrace it.

This does not have to be a deathbed fitness routine either. We've all seen those people! They kill themselves at the gym until they have nothing left, then go to bed and do it all over again the next day. They have zero to offer the world outside of the gym because all their time, energy, and strength is given to the gym. I am not saying you need to be at that level of commitment. While you need to be committed to your goals, your life should still be enjoyable and your habits should be something that can be maintained. You can maintain an intense fifty-minute circuit class; you can't maintain a four-hour cardio marathon with two hours of strength training afterward. So when I say step up your intensity, I do not mean you need to reorganize your entire schedule to fit in three hours of gym time. I simply mean to optimize the time you have dedicated to fitness by changing your workout and increasing its intensity. Remember, everything you do on this journey must be about you and your goals.

Food: This area is tough to evaluate because so many different things can contribute to a plateau. Eating too much, not eating enough, having too many treats, eating on an irregular schedule . . . so many different things! But all of them matter. And it's important to figure out in *your* equation what's not working or needs to be changed. I keep emphasizing "your" because I want you to understand that what works for others might not work for you, and that what worked for me might not work for you. In the same way, this applies to people who constantly feel the need to tell you what you need to be doing and what you should be eating. You can kindly share that your equation is a little different but that you're thankful for their "support."

We all know that one person who shoves their face in all your food and tells you, "That won't help you reach your goals!" or "Should you really be eating that?" Now you can share with them the concept of body equations and your body's individualized equation for reaching your goals. Turn the situation into a teachable moment . . . or drop some knowledge on them that what you're eating is really none of their business. Either method will do!

Eating the right amount—this is a tough concept for some people, especially with society's misconception that twelve hundred calories are what you need to eat if you want to lose weight. That's a ridiculously low number of calories and everyone's body is different. Find the number that works for you. More often than not, people are not losing weight because they are eating too little, not too much. Crazy, right? But it's true, in my experience, at least. You want to be healthy and lose weight, so you eat like Sarah: a day filled with plain rice cakes, wet lettuce salads, and half an orange. That is a recipe for a burnout, a plateau, and a massive binge-eating session when the weekend comes. So find that perfect number for you. What does *your* body need to function at 100 percent? *Healthy weight loss is maintainable; weight loss through crash dieting is not.*

The concept of eating the right amount also includes people who have the opposite problem: those who eat too much. You can eat too much healthy food. Healthy food still has calories. While I have yet to see someone become obese from eating bananas, when you're trying to lose weight, it's important to pay attention to your food sources and to monitor your intake. Find the balance of eating enough while still being able to lose weight. If you eat too little, your body will freak out and plateau, and if you eat too much, your body will store the extra calories and you will also stop seeing results. While it sounds frustrating and complicated to try to figure out your body's equation, keep in mind that this climb is not a race! It's okay to take your time when making your way up Mt. Weight Loss. What matters is that you're moving in the right direction, not how fast you reach the top.

Another food-related factor that can contribute to a plateau is not eating the right things. Not all calories are created equal. One hundred calories from an apple is *not* the same as one hundred calories from a candy bar. While some people like to argue that fifteen hundred calories of fast food is no different from fifteen hundred calories of healthy food . . . it is different. What makes up the calories is important and contributes to how your body breaks down and uses them. You can't outrun a bad diet. Some individuals are blessed with lightning-speed metabolism, and no matter what they eat, they will always have a six-pack under their shirt. Sometimes life just isn't fair! But my guess is you are not that person. And what you eat matters. It matters a lot. Because if you're like me, fifteen hundred calories of fast food will not have the same impact on your body as fifteen hundred calories of healthy food.

If you've never been one to watch the types of food you eat, and you simply pay attention to portion control and count calories . . . can the types of food you're consuming really be the reason you're now at a plateau? Absolutely! Remember, our bodies change. And your body could be telling you, "Hey! I'm not a ten-year-old boy. I need real food. Not fifteen meticulously counted cheese crackers." Think about what you're eating. It might be within the numerical equation your body responds well to, but now the type of food might need to be upgraded. A thousand pounds of dirt do not hold the same value as a thousand pounds of gold. Calories work in a similar way. What are you feeding your body, gold or dirt?

Eating the right amount? Check. Eating the right kinds of food? Check. So what's left to evaluate for possible food contributors to a plateau? Are you eating on a regular basis? You might be the type of person who "forgets" to eat during the day. And I will be honest, that concept is completely alien to me. I look forward to waking up in the morning to eat breakfast. My morning bowl of oatmeal is one of my favorite things, and while I'm eating oatmeal, I'm already looking forward to my mid-morning snack. I love food. I think about eating all the time. I don't "forget" to eat. But some people do. And then when they get home they are hit with a rush of "*I'm starving!*" And then they consume a day's worth of calories in one sitting.

Our bodies are similar to a machine; if you keep the machine well oiled (fed), it will continue to run at optimum speed. When you reduce the frequency of oiling, it does not run as smoothly. Your body will reduce the speed at which it breaks down food. So then when you eat a large amount of food in one sitting, your body will run at a slow and clunky pace. Keep your body functioning at optimum speed by eating the right things frequently and on a good schedule. This will also help reduce those *"I'm starving!"* moments.

Focus: Are you building habits and routines that will get you closer to your goals? Are you actively engaged in creating healthy habits? Are you feeding your healthy habits, or simply restricting your unhealthy habits? Simply restricting habits does not work. You have to replace those habits. Think of your eating habits as a toddler. Toddlers are busy, moody, and unpredictable. They always need to be moving and have something to keep them engaged. You can't simply tell a toddler to stop doing something; you have to redirect them to a more appropriate behavior. Otherwise, they will continue to engage in the undesirable behavior until they move on to something else. You can't say, "Don't do that," and expect them to listen . . . A toddler will do whatever they want. But if you teach or show them something they *can* do instead, the problem behavior will more than likely go away.

Your eating habits work the same way. It's not just a matter of stopping unhealthy behavior, you have to replace the bad behavior with a better alternative. Otherwise, your toddler-like eating habits will make their way back out and you will throw a colossal tantrum in the form of unhealthy eating. Don't be a toddler. *Focus* on replacing those behaviors and actually creating a strategic plan that will help you achieve your goals. You can't expect to successfully reach the top of Mt. Weight Loss with a "whatever happens, happens" mentality. That will leave you stranded, upset, and losing the same five pounds over and over again. Move with a purpose and be focused.

Organization: Are you planning and setting yourself up for success? Scheduling times for workouts and prepping your meals so you don't cave in to whatever food you lay eyes on first? Organization is a critical component to your journey. If you're unorganized, you will plateau. You will stop seeing results. And you might be in this situation right now. Maybe you started out strongly, but now that you've "got the hang of things" you no longer put the same amount of effort into organizing your weekly and daily schedules. This mentality is a recipe for a plateau. The more you engage in healthy behaviors, the more likely they will become second nature to you. Organizing should be one of those healthy behaviors.

I've been living my healthy life for seven years now and I still take time to plan and schedule my week. I take time to organize my weekly schedule and I still use menus to help me plan for the week. At the start of every week, I write out what *all* my meals will be, even snacks! I write them out and then create a grocery shopping list according to the meals I've selected for the week. This will keep me focused and organized when I enter the grocery store. The grocery store is one of those places you do not want to enter without a plan!

It can be easy to slack on organization when you begin to feel, "I've got this healthy eating stuff down." But you can't slack on preparation. If you're like me, the majority of your life was spent being overweight, and you can't simply ignore your history. I'm healthy because I'm actively choosing to engage in a healthy lifestyle; it does not come naturally for me. I created it and continue to develop it. I make a conscious decision to make healthy choices every single day. Now what did become easier throughout my journey was my ability to make those healthy choices. When you first start your journey (this might be where you are right now) every single healthy food option is a daily struggle. You engage in a mental battle between your desire to eat unhealthfully and your longing to reach your weight-loss goals. Every time you walk into the staff lounge and see a plate of cupcakes, you struggle to keep your hands off of them. Everyone experiences this to some degree—you're not alone! And I can assure you that it does become easier to overcome the temptations of the dessert menu. You do get stronger the more you feed your healthy side. What I am trying to ensure you understand is that you can't ignore where you've been and where you currently are. You have to continue to develop your healthy-habit mind-set. You have to be intentional in developing your habits and organizing your day.

Organization applies to more than just food. You also need to be intentional with your workouts. I once heard a great concept that I added to my own mind-set regarding my workout schedule: treat your workouts like a meeting where you're the boss. Bosses don't miss scheduled meetings. At the start of every week organize your weekly exercise schedule. It can be easy to slack on your workouts when the results start to slow down. But this is the time you need to kick it up even more! So if you're experiencing a plateau right now, think about how many rest days you took this week, or how often you skipped a workout because you "just didn't feel like it today." Now don't get me wrong, rest days are super important! That is actually the next area I am going to address. But it can be easy to take too many "rest days" when you start to feel burned out and underwhelmed with your progress. And too many rest days can lead to a plateau.

I understand the burnout feeling. You've been working incredibly hard, waking up early, saying no to all the mouthwatering treats you get offered. Eating salad when you've been dreaming about something fried for weeks. Reaching for an apple when there is a crunchy bowl of chips on display. Sticking to your containers of prepped food at work or school, even though the pizza aroma in the air has you breaking out in a cold sweat. I get it! I've been there. I've been saying no to my dad's *amazing* chicken wings at every family gathering for the past seven years! Those things are so dang good I still dream about them! They're one of the very few non-vegan treats I get cravings for. So I get it. I know it's hard. But any goal worth crushing is going to require some grit. The decision for me to go vegan was the best choice I ever made for my health, but that doesn't mean I don't dream of my previous favorite foods. I will always have an inner part of me that loves junk food.

So if you had to critically evaluate your own organization in the areas of food and exercise . . . how would you do? Would you rate yourself highly on a scale of staying organized and purposeful with your goals and food prep, or would you say that you might need some improvement in this area?

Rest: There are two types of rest-day-related factors that can cause a plateau. There are the individuals who never take a breather to save their life. And then you have the individuals who rest more days than they work. Both can hinder your progress and prevent you from reaching your goals. And I can tell you from experience both situations will halt your progress.

As a group fitness instructor, I get paid to exercise. There was even a time when I was teaching five classes a week and attempting to complete my own personal workouts on the side. Now some instructors "supervise" when they teach; this means they walk around the studio while they lead the class verbally and correct form. This can be an effective technique for instructors to catch their breath or a way for them to still teach while maybe feeling a bit under the weather. Instructors all have those moments! When they can't find a substitute but are still just too sick to go all out while teaching, they "supervise" class rather than participate.

To be honest with you—I'm not a supervising kind of instructor. My style of teaching is that if I'm going to expect you to give your all, I need to model the expected behavior and give my all to you. Nothing irritates me more than an instructor shouting out commands while standing at the back of the room with zero beads of sweat on their body. If you're in my class, we are all sweating. If you're gasping for air, *I'm* gasping for air. I don't just lead you through a workout, I join you. I take breaks because I'm tired or I need to correct form. I don't take breaks because I don't feel like doing the work.

At one point in time I was teaching five classes a week and completing my own personal workouts on top of that. And I was also a full-time graduate student. My life was in constant go-mode. I was up early for class and stayed up late because one of my fitness classes wasn't over until after nine p.m. While coffee has and always will be my blood type, it is not a substitute for sleep. There were some days when I was able to squeeze in a power nap between my responsibilities, but again, there is no substitute for a good night's sleep. Plus, who has time for a solid eight hours of sleep when you have mounds of homework to complete?

Although my schedule was demanding, that did not stop my healthy eating habits. By that point in my journey my healthy food habits had become a solid routine. So if I was dedicated to my workouts and had solid healthy eating habits, why did my progress stop? And why did I stop seeing progress on the scale? Because I never took complete rest days. I never focused on developing healthy recovery habits, such as aiming for a full night of sleep and giving my body a rest day. A rest day for your body is like a watering day for a garden. It happens only about one to two times a week, but it's critical for the nourishment and growth of the garden. I was working hard, but I was not watering my garden.

So if you're facing a plateau, when was the last time you watered your garden? Are you getting enough sleep at night? Are you taking one to two rest days a week? It can be hard to justify rest days, I get it! You want to bring your A-game every single day because your goals are so close. Or you don't want to risk backsliding into old habits, so you focus hard on keeping your gym-game strong. But now your body is tired. And tired bodies are stressed bodies. And stressed is not healthy.

It can be easy to overdo it when you're just getting started, like Sarah sprinting full speed on the treadmill. You have so much motivation the first day that when the fitness gates open up for the race you head out with *all* the strength training and cardio goals in mind. You lift all the weights! Eat all the greens! Drink all the water! Run all the miles! Your warm-up is done with a marathon mentality. Is this a bad thing? It can be. Motivation is great! But exercising beyond your fitness abilities can lead to injury, fatigue, and a case of DOMS (delayed-onset muscle soreness) so severe you can't walk right for the rest of the week. And *that* is not healthy.

No pain, no gain? Sure, but you can't make any gains if you're experiencing so much pain that you can't straighten your arms enough to comb your hair! And that is coming from personal experience. I once had a case of DOMS so ruthless that I had to call for Brea to come help me remove my sports bra . . . not a proud moment. We laughed about it, but in all seriousness, my body was in a grim state of pain and stress. Your body deserves sleep and rest. Evaluate your rest. Planned rest days are just as important as your workouts.

Time: Are you rushing the process? Change takes time, so show patience. Change also takes dedication. Are you committing enough time to reach your goals? Rushing the process is something that not only can cause a plateau, but also can cause defeat. You set out on the incredible mission to completely transform your life, your habits, and your health. And that takes a bit more time than a few weeks. But you find yourself constantly standing on the scale and picking apart your reflection. You're frustrated when a few days pass and the scale hasn't budged. Your focus shifts from reaching your goals to sprinting to them. Have you ever tried to sprint up a mountain? I would guess that most experienced hikers don't head out with a goal to reach the top the fastest. Hikers set out with a goal to reach the top safely and enjoy the hike on the way up.

Your journey up Mt. Weight Loss has to work the same way. It doesn't matter how fast you get to the top; what matters is that you arrive there safely and with the tools needed to *maintain* your healthy life. If you're too focused on sprinting, you might lose your footing and slip and fall. Or you might be so focused on the sprint that you miss the opportunity to develop the healthy habits needed to continue the climb up the mountain range beyond Mt. Weight Loss, the abundant mountain range of Weight Maintenance.

I remember one day I was sharing my frustration with my sister and my mom about how it had been two weeks and I was still stuck at the same weight (at this point I was around 155 pounds). My sister said, "Sharee, look how far you have come, though! You seem so focused on losing more weight that you're not really appreciating how far you've already come." My initial reaction was to argue and become defensive. I made some snide comment about how I was enjoying my journey. But later on I realized that she was right! I was so focused on the end result that I had lost sight of the day-to-day enjoyment of being healthy. My journey had morphed into a numbers game and I was stuck playing the game with the scale. And I hated that! That's not me! That's not how I wanted to look back and think of my journey. I had worked too hard to be stuck playing a game with the scale.

And *you* have worked too hard and will work too hard to be stuck playing the same scale game. Is the scale important? Yes, in the sense that you should aim to attain a healthy weight range. But that's about it. When you start focusing on your health, your eating habits, your sleeping habits, and your fitness, the scale will take care of itself. So where is your focus? On the important things that will help you continue to live a healthy life beyond Mt. Weight Loss? Or are you stuck playing a game with the scale and sprinting to the top, so focused on the time and the numbers that you can't even allow yourself to enjoy the journey?

But what about the opposite time-related factor? You're so focused on sleep that you can't possibly spend thirty minutes a day walking. You view rest days as being so important that you have six of them every week. Well, at this point, you're not watering your garden, you're drowning it. When I first started my journey, that was me. I would go work out with my mom one time a week and call it good—and I use the words "work out" liberally. I would go to the gym and move things around . . . but I had zero focus, intensity, or purpose. I had the desire to lose weight. But I did not have the dedication. Simply going through the motions will not get results. Your heart and mind need to be on the journey too, not just your body.

One of the very first gyms I ever joined was an all-female gym. The gym was designed in a way so that all you had to do was show up and go through a circuit of machines a few times, and that was your workout. There were motivational success stories on the walls about weight loss and body transformations. And I was determined to have a similar story worth featuring on a wall. My mom and I were regular attendees. I knew all the employees and would chat with the other regular attendees. It was a fun and supportive atmosphere. But while other people were achieving their goals, my weight was not budging. It came down to my lack of focus. I was not moving with a purpose. I was not focused on raising my heart rate and breaking a sweat. I thought that by simply walking into a gym, my effort in being there would warrant my weight to drop. Well, I hate to break it to you, but fat does not go away simply because you walk into a gym. Gyms are not holy water symbolically flung onto the evil fat layers on your body. If you want a hot body, you're going to have to do more than the elliptical at a leisurely pace for thirty-five minutes. Losing weight is hard work. It's not impossible, but it is hard.

The time you dedicate to your goals must reflect the size of your goals. If you have big goals, your time commitment should be big. Genius, right? Evaluate your E.F.F.O.R.T.: Exercise, Food, Focus, Organization, Rest, and Time. If you're not seeing results, or your progress has stopped, you might be lacking in one or more of these areas.

Whether or not you're experiencing a plateau right now, it is beneficial to evaluate your E.F.F.O.R.T. to identify shortcomings you may experience in the future. Either way, it can help you redirect and refocus your mission. Now for some critical self-evaluation time. How is your E.F.F.O.R.T.?

Exercise: Are you keeping up with a routine? Are you switching things up to keep it challenging?

____

____

____

Food: Are you eating enough, eating the right things, and eating often? Are you avoiding the junk?

____

____

____

Focus: Are you building habits and routines that will get you closer to your goals?

____

____

____

Organization: Are you planning and setting yourself up for success? Are you scheduling times for workouts? Are you dedicating time to prep your weekly meals?

Rest: Are you allowing your body the rest it needs? Are you watering your garden weekly? Or are you taking too many rest days, drowning your garden?

Time: Are you rushing the process? Change takes time, so are you showing patience? Change also takes dedication. Are you committing enough time to reach your goals?

7

The Magic Twelve Hundred

Twelve hundred. That's the magic number for weight loss, right? If you eat only twelve hundred calories a day all your weight-loss dreams will come true and you will be prancing around with your dream body in no time! If you eat twelve hundred calories your wildest weight-loss dreams will become a reality and your body will radiate health and bikini-body readiness. There is nothing you can't accomplish when you begin to eat twelve hundred calories daily! Well . . . that's what uniformed and poorly written magazine articles will tell you. I am not a nutritionist. I am not a personal trainer. I am a certified and practicing school psychologist with a passion for and teaching background in group fitness. So this information I am about to share is not coming from a book. It's coming from my personal experience of losing half my body weight.

Walking to school in the morning wasn't so bad; it gave me an opportunity to play through the fence with the baby cows that lived on the farm near my house. And sometimes I would see Mrs. Jones out in her garden pruning her magnificent flowerbeds. Every couple of weeks she would deliver flowers to the houses on the street. The bouquets were stunning and were the centerpiece of my family's dining table.

"Hi, Mrs. Jones," I shouted one morning on my way to school. She smiled and waved as I got on the bus. However, something stuck out to me that morning; Mrs. Jones was standing by her gardening beds, but she wasn't pruning anything. She was just walking around the flowers shaking her head. I didn't think anything of it, apart from that it was odd. But after all, she was kind of elderly.

A couple weeks went by and I noticed that we didn't have any new flowers on our table for dinner. "Mom," I said, "why don't we have any new flowers? Is Mrs. Jones okay?"

"She's fine, dear," my mom said. "Mrs. Jones stopped by earlier today. I guess she's having problems with her flowers this year. Maybe in a couple weeks we will have some new flowers." She shrugged. "But I do have some gardening tools I need to return to her. You can drop them off on your way to school and ask her about her flowers. I sure do miss how they lighten up the whole kitchen." I nodded my head and finished my dinner.

The following morning I left for school a few minutes early to ensure enough time to stop to talk to Mrs. Jones. As I approached her house her lawn looked gloomy and lifeless. My mouth hung wide as visions of her previously magnificent gardens were washed away at the sight of this flower graveyard. I saw her kneeling on the other side of the lawn. "Mrs. Jones!" I shouted. "What happened to your flowers? Everything is dead! All the flowers are wilted! What happened?!" I gasped.

Mrs. Jones looked up with tears in her eyes and said, "My garden was overrun with weeds so I stopped watering it. I thought it would kill the weeds . . . and it did. But it took the good with them. Now all my flowers—all my hard work—are gone!" Tears streamed down her face as she gazed at what were once magnificent flowerbeds.

When your method for losing weight is eating less than your body needs, it's as if you're withholding water from a garden in an attempt to kill the weeds. You lose the good with the bad. You cannot solely target the fat on your body by means of starvation. You cannot create a healthy life by unhealthy means. Water the garden. Feed your body. Now, I have never heard of an avid and experienced gardener starving their flowerbeds, but I have heard of people starving to reach their goals and eating less than their bodies need. Twelve hundred calories are not enough. This "magic" number for weight loss will destroy your metabolism. You will lose the good. It's not a matter of "if," but a matter of when. Consuming only twelve hundred calories is not healthy and it's not maintainable.

But how? People lose weight all the time eating twelve hundred calories. Yes, they do! But what happens when they resume eating the number of calories that a grown adult is supposed to eat (twelve hundred calories is the recommended amount for a six-year-old child)? They gain their weight back. *How you lose the weight is how your body learns to maintain it.* Twelve hundred calories is crash-dieting in numerical form. Twelve hundred calories is a haphazard piece of information littering magazines that promote "Lose 10 Pounds in 10 Minutes!" bogusness. It doesn't work and it's not practical. If you really stop to think about what you're putting your body through when you eat only twelve hundred calories, you will see why it doesn't work.

So what does eating twelve hundred calories actually do? Our bodies have adapted to survive based on the environment we live in. If you continually eat less than your body needs to function fully, will your body continue to function at 100 percent? No. That's like expecting a car to complete a road trip that requires a full tank of gas, but filling the tank only halfway. The car will stop. And so will our bodies. Our bodies will be forced to decide what can be sacrificed in order to maintain productivity. If you give your body only 65 percent of the nutrients it needs,it will operate only at 65 percent productivity. It's not rocket science. I don't need a background in nutrition to tell you that your body will not run on six hundred calories a day simply because you decided that it should.

Your body will start to slow down. Your metabolism will decrease to glacier speed. And if you're trying to lose weight, you want the opposite to happen. You want to improve your metabolism, not slow it down. You want your body to quickly burn through food (which is our bodies' fuel), not slowly break it down. Your cognitive speed will decrease. Your immune system will be compromised. Your hair and nails will dull. Who needs shiny hair and nails when your body is under the impression that it's starving? If you are a woman, you risk stopping your menstrual cycle. Your cortisol levels will skyrocket, and chronic stress is never good. Exercise? Yeah, right! Your body is *starving*—do you think you will have any energy to run a few miles? The slightest amount of exercise will leave you feeling exhausted. When you feel exhausted and sluggish . . . is that going to help motivate you to get to the gym? When you feel like crap you don't bring your A-game.

But what about losing weight? Yes, initially you will. Your body will flush out water and various toxins. But after you lose water weight, you will begin to lose weight painfully slowly. And the moment you begin to eat the amount your body actually needs, you will gain weight. Your body will start to realize, "Hmm, I have not received enough food recently . . . Maybe all the food is gone! I'm going to starve to death unless I begin to store everything that enters me!" So you literally become walking food storage. Your body does not burn the food you eat. It stores it. You will gain weight easier because your body is convinced you're starving . . . And honestly, you are.

Still not convinced, right? How many people do you see who are able to eat twelve hundred calories on a regular basis and not complain about needing to lose the same ten pounds over and over again? They reach their goal weight, then go back to eating "normally," and they gain weight back! You cannot be healthy if you're starving your flowerbed. Water your garden. Eat like an adult. Eat enough. And eat the right things. How you lose the weight is how your body learns to maintain it. I keep making that statement, but what does it actually mean? What does eating to maintain your weight loss actually entail?

It means that your climb up Mt. Weight Loss must include learning what a healthy lifestyle is and what a healthy lifestyle will look like for you. What good is losing fifty-plus pounds if you never learn how to keep it off?! If all you do is eat rice cakes and drink fifteen gallons of water for eight weeks . . . what does that teach you about life? Are you going to follow this super-restrictive diet for the rest of your life? If the answer is no, then the method you're using is not maintainable. And you will be one of those people constantly gaining and losing weight. That is why it's so incredibly important to pick a healthy eating lifestyle you *enjoy*. Because it's going to be a lifestyle you will have to maintain if you ever want to be a success story. If your diet has an expiration date, then weight gain is inevitable. If you can't wait to "go back to eating normal food," then weight gain is inevitable. *Diets do not work. Lifestyle changes work.* You can live in denial all you want—but the scale won't lie.

Follow that twelve-hundred-calorie diet for eight weeks. Reach your goal of losing ten pounds. And then see how long it takes you to gain it back. I'm not negative, I'm being honest. You have the opportunity to be a success story, to reach your goals, to conquer Mt. Weight Loss! But what it takes is dedication to creating a healthy life. Not a crash diet. Not a pill. Not a detox. A thoughtful and you-centered plan will help shape and create the healthy life you want to live. This is your life—you should be able to enjoy it! What is there to enjoy about six hundred calories a day of rice cakes and plain oatmeal? What is there to look forward to when you're so tired you can't appreciate your life because you're constantly emotionally and physically drained?

Weight loss is not magic, it's science. And you just need to find the equation that is right for your body. But I can assure you, twelve hundred calories is not the equation for a lasting, healthy, and weight-maintaining life. Our bodies need a specific number of calories to maintain their vital functions (i.e., heartbeat, breathing, organs, etc.). All the things our bodies do require energy, and our bodies' source of fuel is calories. When you begin to reduce the number of calories you consume, your body will be forced to limit productivity. When you exercise, you steal calories from your body that otherwise would go toward everyday regular functions. Those stolen calories need to be replenished. You need to eat enough for your body to function while you maintain a healthy, active life. Find that balance between eating enough and not overeating. Remember, weight loss is science, not magic.

So now you might be thinking, *Okay, got it! Eat enough! This process is science, not magic, blah, blah, blah . . . We get it! But what are the right things to eat? What types of foods are healthy?!* Diet culture shoves all these different methods in our faces: paleo, Raw till 4, juicing, vegan, low carb, low calorie, and a host of other food trends and "lifestyles." An obscene amount of information is relentlessly flooding our brains until we have absolutely no idea what a "normal" healthy person actually eats! You just want to lose weight! Why is it so hard to find solid information on what you can and cannot eat? How do you know what is right for you with so many different opinions out there?!

Trust me. I get how confusing it is to shift through the infinite opinions, articles, diet books, and self-proclaimed nutrition and weight-loss experts. But the truth is, there is no one-size-fits-all when it comes to specific diets and ways of eating. What works for me might not work for you. What worked for your friend might not work for you. What does fit everyone is healthy eating. But healthy will look different in terms of lifestyle and food choices.

I'm vegan; my husband is not. Are we both healthy? Yes. My dad tends to eat low carb and my mom follows portion control and limits her junk food. Are they both healthy? Yes. I know people who have lost incredible amounts of weight following a low-carb diet. Would that work for me? No. But it worked for them and they are healthy. The point is, you have to make your food lifestyle about you. You have to make your food habits about you. Don't feel pressured to follow a way of eating that would never work for you. Everyone deserves to live a healthy life, but that doesn't mean you have to become vegan and live off of dates and blended bananas for the rest of your life. What needs to be replaced are the unhealthy eating habits you identified earlier, those habits that are preventing you from reaching your goals. In order for me to replace my unhealthy eating habits I had to limit my opportunities to eat certain foods by adopting a vegan lifestyle.

So what does healthy food look like? Whole grains, lean proteins, fruits, veggies, and healthy fats. Those are the recommended food groups that will give our bodies all the nutrition, vitamins, and minerals that we need. *But* the ratio and the amount you eat from each group will depend on what healthy looks like for you. If you want me to give you a meal guide that will guarantee weight loss, you're reading the wrong book. I don't do that. I don't sell meal plans. I share practical advice that I learned along my journey and things I wish I had learned sooner. I share them in a way that motivates *you* to create a healthy meal plan and get started on your own personal journey.

There are lots of different paths up Mt. Weight Loss. I want to help you find the motivation to choose the right one. I won't choose the path for you. By taking control of your own eating habits and understanding the habits that are impacting your health, you are that much closer to reaching your goals.

My background and work in education always has me saying, "Show me the data." Whenever there is talk about changing a child's placement or anything related to change, data is always the reason behind the movement and the evidence to support the change. *You* can use data to track your progress too. If you're not sure what style of eating will work for you, be your own experiment. Keep a food journal that tracks your daily intake but also records how you're feeling, your daily exercise, and your stats (e.g., weight, body measurements, etc.). If you ran a few miles that night, how did you feel afterward? Did you feel ready to take on the world when you woke up this morning, or did this way of eating leave you feeling drained and irritable? Give yourself three to four weeks to see how your body responds. Again, it's not a race! It's okay to try different things out to see what works and what's not for you. This is only the rest of your life we are talking about. So take your time; carefully collect the evidence to support your decision to stick with a certain way of eating. Be picky and be persistent.

Take a moment to think about what healthy might look like for you. Are you considering trying a different way of eating, such as low carb or vegan? Is it practical? Is it you-centered? Below are some common diets and ways of eating that people adopt for their healthy life. See if one interests you and try it out. If you don't see one you want to try—because again, these are just ideas, not the be-all and end-all of weight loss—create your own eating lifestyle and types of food goals you want to achieve.

Clean Eating: This is pretty basic and just a general way to describe healthy eating. A clean-eating lifestyle is high in vegetables, fruits, whole grains, lean meats, fish, low-fat dairy, eggs, nuts, and healthy fats, and low in processed foods, refined sugar, and processed grains. This is essentially the staple description of a successful method of healthy eating. From this description, people create subcategories of eating and fine-tune their personal preferences, such as eliminating dairy or opting to not eat meat. The ratios of food groups are changed depending on personal preference as well. But essentially, healthy eating will generally encompass the idea of whole foods over processed foods. Some people are guided by their morals to eliminate food groups (e.g., vegans abstain from eating meat in an effort to raise awareness of animal cruelty and the meat industry) and some people eliminate food groups for health reasons. Whatever your reasons are, it's important to understand that this is a personal choice and people will have varying ideas on what "healthy" means. Just remember that what matters is that you're happy with your eating lifestyle and that your eating style reflects you as a person.

Low Carb: Carbohydrates are a main nutrient for our bodies and also arguably one of our bodies' most important sources of fuel. Our bodies break down the carbohydrates we consume into glucose (sugar) that can then be used for energy. When too many carbohydrates are consumed (or too much of anything, for that matter; fat and protein are in the same boat), or all the "energy" consumed is not used, our bodies will store the excess as fat. Without going into super-science and super-nutrition mode, when you reduce the body's fuel supply—in this case, the amount of carbs you eat—your body will be forced to use its stored fuel supplies. And if you have a lot of extra stored fuel (fat) on your body, your body will begin to break it down.

Arguably, simply reducing calories will have the same effects and your body will break down stored fat, but some people have a lot of success with the low-carb approach. This is similar to how I have had great success with a vegan diet. Were the eliminated animal by-products what resulted in my weight loss, or was it the fact that I began to eat more fruits and vegetables and had less room for junk food? Does limiting or eliminating carbs help with weight loss, or does the overall attention to food intake? Either way, it's important to find a style that works for you.

The amount of carbohydrates will vary depending on the person and their individual preferences. Some people will aim for below twenty grams of carbs and other people consider low carb to be around one hundred grams a day. Ultimately, you will have to find what works for your body and what you respond to. Low-carb diets center on dairy products (typically full fat to avoid added sugar and carbs), meat, eggs, fish, low-carb fruits such as grapefruit, low-carb green vegetables, nuts, and seeds. Foods that are avoided include sugary fruit, colorful and starchy vegetables, beans, whole grains, breads and pastas, oats, and highly processed foods.

Low carb is something that works very well for my dad but does not work well for me. If you enjoy eggs and turkey bacon in the morning and can live without peanut butter and toast, this might be something for you to look into. Again, it's your journey! Make it enjoyable!

Carb-Cycling: This is similar to low carb except you have days when you aim to eat a high amount of carbs and you have days when you eat a low amount. Theamount of carbs you eat will vary depending on personal preference and what your body responds to. Carb-cycling is a common practice amongst people trying to lose weight. You might have two days of low carb followed by one day of high carb, and then another two days of low carb, etc. A pro of carb-cycling is that it is easy to modify for everyday life circumstances, such as going to restaurants and family outings. But ultimately, any method or style of eating can be modified when you eat out; it just depends on how much thought you're willing to put into it.

Low-carb days will follow your typical low-carb diet: green vegetables, eggs, dairy, fish, lean meats, nuts, and seeds. And high-carb days can consist of fruits, whole grains, oats, colorful vegetables, and proteins. Carb-cycling is something that will require planning on a continual basis, including thoughtful meal planning and purposeful grocery shopping (although, if you're eating healthfully, meal planning and conscientious grocery shopping will be a part of your week regardless). What is different about carb-cycling compared to other types of eating is that you will be shopping for two distinct types of eating styles. So if this is an eating option you want to try, seek out additional resources to help guide you. Healthy eating will always have benefits! So don't panic if you're not sure what route you want to go; just try things out and see what works. But again, take your time. It's not a race.

Vegan: This is my soul-mate eating style, but that does not mean it's right for everyone! A vegan or plant-based diet includes vegetables, whole grains, fruits, plant-based proteins (tofu, tempeh, etc.), nuts, nut butters, and plant-based dairy products (soy, almond, coconut, etc.). A vegan diet does not include eggs, dairy products, meat, or fish. Anything that comes from an animal is not consumed on a vegan diet. Some variations of the vegan diet include eating a vegan diet certain days of the week (similar to carb-cycling) or eating vegan until dinnertime or a particular time of the day.

What is important is that you find something that works for you and something that is maintainable! Having the ability to eat at restaurants without monumental complications is important to me, and it might be something that you need to consider when deciding what healthy eating will look like for you. Dre is not vegan, so when we go out on date nights, we don't stick to vegan-only restaurants. Sometimes he wants a burger and other times he wants pasta. And I can manage to find enjoyable things to eat that suit my preferences at different types of restaurants. You don't want to feel isolated and alone when it comes to eating. That will not lead to happiness and health. It will lead to you feeling frustrated and going back to eating "normally." Remember, if "normal" is a word you find yourself using to describe how other people eat, then you have not yet found an eating style right for you. How you eat should be "normal" in your eyes.

Raw: Raw diets are increasing in popularity because a lot of celebrity and inspirational figures are releasing raw cookbooks and continually updating their social media accounts with raw-food information—not to mention the mouthwatering recipes that flood social media outlets on a daily basis. Raw is a plant-based and vegan diet where all the food is consumed "raw" and uncooked. Produce can be chilled, frozen, blended, chopped, ground, etc. But the food cannot be cooked using a heat source or other processing methods. Fruits, vegetables, and raw nuts are what this diet consists of. Refined sugar, salt, oils, processed baking ingredients, and grains are avoided.

The only hesitation I have with a raw diet is that it can pack a lot of calories. Healthy calories, absolutely! But many of the recipes include four or five bananas with cups of dates and blended soaked nuts. When you're trying to lose weight, calories matter, plain and simple. Even healthy calories! Your body will not burn four thousand extra calories because you decided that it should. Now, will an extra banana on top of your calorie goals halt your progress? It's doubtful. But consume an extra five bananas every day (that's over five hundred calories in bananas alone), and that can add up at the end of the week.

My body would not respond well on a raw diet, *but* that does not mean that yours won't. Again, collect your data. Track your progress and find what your body responds to. And also ask yourself if you can maintain this lifestyle. How you lose the weight is how your body will learn to maintain it. If raw allows you to reach your goal weight, raw is what it will take to maintain your weight. If you have been wondering what it would be like to make your own almond milk and nut butters, maybe the raw diet is for you.

It's important to keep in mind that raw diets should also consist of vegetables. Many raw-food lovers share creative recipes that center on fruits, nuts, and seeds—which is great. Who wouldn't want to eat banana, cocoa, and cashew ice cream for every meal? But vegetables are important too and shouldn't be left out. There are also raw forms of protein that you can purchase, and other raw ingredients from local grocery stores to help make the transition easier. Just like with any diet, you want to make sure you're eating balanced and nutrient-filled meals. The process will take practice and planning to ensure your body is receiving all the nutrients and vitamins that it needs. Be patient with the learning process but be diligent in your planning. Far too often, individuals pull a Sarah and jump into a lifestyle of eating without educating themselves fully. As a result, they end up with health complications because their body was not receiving enough nutrients. Be smart and be responsible; it should be common sense to know that your body needs more than bananas and dates to function.

If you're intrigued about the raw-food lifestyle, but you're not sure if it's for you, maybe try it for a few weeks and see what you think. Try a two- or three-week raw diet challenge. Get some friends or family members to try it with you. What a great way to create a circle of support and shared dietary "struggles." I'm not a fan or supporter of detoxes, but a raw-food challenge would be a good way to jump-start a healthy eating mind-set. It's a natural way to detox, by simply not eating junk food anymore!

Paleo: Often referred to as the "caveman diet," it's essentially the opposite of a vegan diet. The idea is that you eat what our ancestors had available to them. If bacon burgers are your thing, this might be for you, minus the bun and the cheese. The paleo diet consists primarily of fish, grass-fed and pasture-raised meats, eggs, vegetables, fruit, fungi, roots, and nuts. It excludes grains, legumes, dairy products, potatoes, refined salt and sugar, and processed oils. Some people opt to follow this diet a few days a week or challenge themselves to a month of paleo eating. But again, make sure you pick a lifestyle that your body responds to and that you learn from.

Challenges are great! But after the challenge you want to make sure you have a game plan to continue your success. If eating meat is your "thing" but you need more structure in your life, paleo is a popular lifestyle of eating. However, balance is also needed, as with any lifestyle. You can't eat bacon and red meat for every meal and neglect vegetables. You might find bacon to be mouthwatering, but bacon will not replace the nutrients found in vegetables. As with any lifestyle, it's important to establish balanced eating habits (i.e., protein, fat, iron, calcium, etc.), and it's important to educate yourself on ways to ensure a balanced diet. Think of the food pyramid. Are you eating all the categories? It's not about the specific foods in them (e.g., grains or diary), but more so the nutrients found in those sources of food. Are you eating in a way that ensures you get all the nutrients your body needs? Calories, sodium, processed ingredients, fat content, etc. . . . All these things matter for weight loss. So when exploring various ways of eating, keep in mind that "clean eating" is the general idea, and within that, narrow down the possibilities. With so many different paths to take to reach the top of Mt. Weight Loss, it's okay to take your time to decide which path will work best for you.

Vegetarian and Pescatarian: These two diets are not 100 percent similar but they are related enough to be grouped into one category. A vegetarian does not eat fish or meat; a pescatarian eats fish but not meat. Both eat dairy, eggs, grains, nuts, legumes, fats, processed foods, refined foods, etc. The diet can be modified to your preferences. You can be a vegetarian who does not eat dairy, or you can be a dairy- and egg-free pescatarian. This is about you and what you feel works for you. I was not successful as a vegetarian; I ate cheese and crackers 24/7, and that was not healthy! Find your balance. Track your daily intake, exercise, and make sure you're eating grains, vegetables, fruit, and meat-free protein. Create a healthy, balanced diet that you feel confident will get you to your goals. Find a lifestyle that will help you replace those unhealthy eating habits that are holding you back. Veganism made it easier for me to replace my unhealthy habits, but it still took work. I could no longer eat fried chicken, but I could still purchase fried foods. I still had to learn how to replace those unhealthy habits, and you will too.

Low Carb, High Fat (LCHF): A LCHF diet is focused on consuming few carbs and higher amounts of fat. Though similar to a low-carb diet, it places more emphasis on higher fat content. LCHF diets include fish, eggs, meat, low-carb vegetables, and healthy fats. Foods that are avoided include bread, rice, potatoes, oats, grains, sugar, starchy vegetables, and most fruits.

High Carb, Low Fat (HCLF): The complete opposite of the diet mentioned above, this is a diet rich in fruits and high-carb root vegetables, such as potatoes. Oftentimes HCLF individuals are also vegan or vegetarian, but this is not a requirement. From my experience, HCLF individuals tend to eat more on the raw side and consume lots of smoothies, banana-based meals, and high-carb vegetable meals. As with any method of eating, if you're aiming to lose weight, it's important to ensure you're eating enough and eating the right portions. It's easy to both overeat and undereat when consuming primarily fruits, nuts, and vegetables.

There are so many options out there, each with its own pros and cons. Again, find an eating style that seems like something you would be successful at. And if you're unsure, try a few out. Don't worry if you're switching around every three to four weeks, as this is your life and health we are talking about. You're not changing a pair of socks! This process will take time. It might take experimenting with two or three different eating styles until you figure out what your body responds well to. And that is okay! Take all the time you need to establish your own eating style. Healthy eating is healthy eating.

What diet will work for you? Take this time to complete a list of questions that might help you identify a way of eating that would work for you on your journey and beyond.

- What clean-eating area will be the hardest for you to follow during your journey? Clean-eating concepts include unprocessed whole foods, lean meats and meat alternatives, whole grains, fruits, vegetables, limited refined sugar, and low-fat dairy items and dairy-free alternatives.

____

____

____

- What are your favorite foods that follow clean-eating guidelines (i.e., not treat foods like ice cream and cookies)?

____

____

____

- What foods can you not live without (e.g., cheese, chicken, bread, fruit, etc.)?

____

____

____

- What is your biggest food-category weakness (e.g., mine was dairy; all I wanted to eat was cheese or dairy products)?

____

____

____

- Is this food category preventing you from reaching your goals? Can you opt for a healthier version, or do you need to ditch the food group altogether (e.g., I went vegan, which meant no more access to dairy products)?

____

____

____

- What style of eating appeals to you? Are you going to follow the clean-eating guidelines or are you considering trying a more structured way of eating (i.e., vegan, paleo, carb-cycling, etc.)?

____

____

____

- If you want to create your own style of eating, write it out below. What foods will you include? What foods are you going to avoid?

____

____

____

8

Loose Skin, Stretch Marks, and Body Image

This chapter is going to be a little bit different from the others. I am going to tackle specific issues, questions, and topics that I encounter regularly, topics and questions ranging from loose skin and body image to negative individuals. Maybe you have never struggled with these topics, or maybe every single area will hit home for you. We are all on the journey together. So even if you're not experiencing these situations directly, someone around you might be. And at one point, they may need your support and guidance to help them.

It's one sit-up, Sharee, come on! I yelled to myself in my head. But no matter how hard I tried, I couldn't get my body to coordinate the movement of a sit-up. No matter how much I tried to contract my core, it was as if the muscles were dead. My roommate, Brea, was on the workout mat next to me, laughing. It must have been a pretty entertaining sight for her to see. Sharee, the self-proclaimed fitness queen, couldn't complete one sit-up. I was trying not to laugh and to stay focused on flexing my muscles, but nothing worked. I joined Brea on the mat and just laughed with her while the workout DVD continued to play.

I was the one who had wanted this workout program. Late one night, I was doing some homework on my bed when a commercial on TV promoting a martial arts–style fitness program came on. The commercial was so motivating and intriguing that it made me want to get up and exercise that minute! I called Brea into my room and made her watch the whole forty-five-minute segment. She agreed that it looked really fun and like something she would enjoy doing. But I couldn't do the workouts with her. I still had more recovering to do.

Loose Skin: Ten weeks after my tummy-tuck surgery, I was just starting to get back into working out, and still trying to figure out my abdominal muscles. I never knew what loose skin was until I had some. It never occurred to me that loose skin was even a possibility. Once I realized that I had loose skin, I began the process of researching what people do to correct it. Thus began my extensive research into the world of tummy tucks.

If you have never done online research on skin removal surgery, I suggest you keep it that way. The horror stories of what can go wrong and the horrific pictures of people who look as though they've been hacked in half and sewn and stapled back together . . . will leave you traumatized. *Who would voluntarily get a surgery like that?!* I thought to myself. But then I would see the shocking tummy-tuck "before" and "after" photos, with scars that had healed nicely and were barely visible. Maybe I would be able to endure the surgery.

I began to research the procedure and what it would entail. Loose skin is not something that corrects itself. Not everyone will face loose skin. There are plenty of stories where people have lost over a hundred pounds and did not have any loose skin. And there are people who gain fifty pounds during pregnancy and develop loose skin. Loose skin is not something that corrects itself (I've said that twice for those in the back, the judgmental individuals who have negative views of those who have opted for plastic surgery). The appearance of loose skin can improve with strength training and time, depending on a person's age, the amount of time spent being overweight, and genetics. But loose skin does not shrink back and attach to muscles on its own. That's where skin removal surgery comes into play.

There are lots of different types of surgeries, some that include muscle repair if needed, as well as different incision lines, lengths, etc. I didn't know any of this until I had loose skin and began to research what options there are for skin removal. I wasn't unhappy with myself. I was so thrilled and proud of all the hard work I had put into my weight loss. Nothing could hold back my feelings of pride and accomplishment. The reason I elected for skin removal surgery was because honestly, I could. I had the means to move forward with the surgery. I sought out an amazing doctor who had incredible results in previous surgeries. And I opted to have a tummy tuck and thigh lift. A thigh lift is the removal of loose skin from the inner and upper thighs.

Would I have been happy without ever receiving skin removal surgery? Absolutely. So why did I receive it? Because I could afford it. It was within my realm of control. I received my tummy tuck six months before my wedding. My honeymoon to Mexico was the first time I ever wore a bikini on the beach! But my tummy tuck did not bring me happiness. In fact, the recovery just about sent me into a depression. It's a difficult surgery to bounce back from, both mentally and physically. The swelling is so intense that it's called "swell hell" and lasts for months. You gain ten-plus pounds immediately following the surgery because of the amount of swelling you endure. You lose your muscles and endurance because you can't do anything active for at least two months. You're in pain, filled with stitches, and have drain tubes attached to your body. The first time you catch a glimpse of your stitches, you start to question if you made the right choice. I knew I had made the right choice, but when you look as if you're ready to be on the set of a zombie movie, you start to question your life choices!

There was one point when I broke down into tears in the middle of the grocery store while shopping with Dre. All he wanted to know was what I wanted for dinner. But all I could focus on was how swollen I looked and felt, how I was so tired all the time, and how much I missed teaching fitness classes. At the time, I was a full-time graduate student. I had the surgery over spring break and was back in class on day seventeen. Fitness was my stress release, but because of my surgery, I couldn't work out anymore. So as a result, I turned into a puddle of tears at the grocery store, crying on Dre's shoulder as he uncomfortably looked around the store, hoping that no one thought he'd been the one who'd made me cry. Dre wasn't the only one who had to deal with my mood swings. Brea had her share of lots of my late-night tear sessions too, times when I would complain about how none of my clothes fit and how angry I was with my swelling. But it's all part of the process. And for me, it was something that I am grateful I endured. It was worth it. My entire journey was worth it. I have stretch marks. I have scars. But I also have my whole life ahead of me because I'm healthy!

So what if you get loose skin at the end of a journey? So what if you have stretch marks? Are stretch marks and loose skin worse than having a heart attack at the age of forty?! If you're healthy, active, and happy, who is going to care about the condition of your skin and whether or not you have stretch marks? You cannot control your skin elasticity. But you can control your weight. Focus on what you can control.

It's all too easy to fall into a puddle of self-pity when looking at Photoshopped pictures of models and their perfect skin. Just as a piece of advice, I've had a professional photo shoot, and the amount of makeup you wear would hide a fresh bullet wound! Magazines are not real life. Not even the people in the magazines look like the people in the magazines. If you want motivation, go to the gym and people-watch for a gym-crush. Find individuals in real life who can motivate you and encourage you, not computer-generated individuals in magazines with unrealistic beauty standards. I'm not motivated by the girls on the covers of fashion magazines, I'm motivated by my mom, who is the mother of three children and has a killer six-pack that she earned! The girl at the gym who recently crushed a bikini competition motivates me. The women at the beach who rock string bikinis even with stretch marks and cellulite motivate me! Never be ashamed of who you are and what you're fighting for. You will have good days and you will have bad days, but that doesn't mean that the journey is not worth it. Your health is always worth it.

What if you can't afford to ever have skin removal? That is okay! Again, reaching your goals and taking control of your health are more important than loose skin. Loose skin will not ruin your life, unless you let it. I know people who have let the fear of loose skin hold them back from ever trying to reach their goals. And I don't get that. I honestly cannot wrap my mind around that concept. You would rather continue to be unhappy and frustrated with your weight than take charge and lose weight because of the possibility of loose skin? I don't understand how a "what-if" idea can shape your current life and choices. That is beyond me. Please don't be that person. Please do not let the possibility of loose skin prevent you from taking control of your life and your health. If you end up with loose skin, that is okay. And *if* that happens, you will cross that bridge when you get there. Right now your focus should be on creating the best version of you, crushing your goals, and taking control of your health.

If you are a person who has already lost the weight and reached the top of Mt. Weight Loss and now have loose skin, please do not let that make you second-guess your decision to lose weight. While loose skin is not the most exciting thing in the whole entire world, it's certainly not the worst. I rocked a monokini when I had loose skin. I still wore short shorts even with loose skin on my thighs. I busted my butt for my body, and while some parts of me were "loose," other parts of me looked freaking awesome! So I made sure to show those off. I focused on what I could control; that has always been my driving force on my journey. Do not let loose skin hold you back from continuing your life of health and happiness. You have worked too hard to reach your goals to let loose skin continue to bring you down.

A Note to the Negative Nancys: Some people wear their loose skin like a badge of honor. Some individuals take pride in their loose skin and choose to not have it removed. I have my tummy-tuck scar to show the battle I overcame with obesity. It doesn't matter what other people think about *your* body. It matters what you think. So if you're someone who disagrees with plastic surgery, then don't get it. But don't judge people who don't have the same beliefs as you. Everyone is on this journey to be healthy and happy. And that will look different for everyone.

Don't be the body police. *People's bodies are not property to be judged, rated, or valued based on personal opinions.* In today's society, we have this belief that you can say anything you want because it's "your opinion." Absolutely, have an opinion! Have your own ideas, thoughts, and beliefs. But don't justify being a body-shamer, the food police, and the body-image patrol as "your opinion." A body is *not* open to the opinions of anyone other than those of its owner. If you think breast implants are gross, that's your right. Don't get them! If you would never *dare* to have an arm lift, that is your choice! But don't take your ideas and verbally projectile-vomit on everyone within earshot who disagrees with you. People's bodies are not up for debate. If it's not your body, then you have no right to voice an opinion about it.

The first time my weight was insulted by a complete stranger, I didn't feel motivated to lose weight. Their rude comments didn't send me to the grocery store with healthy food on my mind. I wasn't inspired by the stranger who called me a "fat ass" to go to the gym and hit the treadmill. Mean and rude comments do not elicit motivation from people. Laughing at individuals who are overweight will not make them evaluate their food choices. Harassing overweight people will not prompt them to give up soda. Those types of comments are rude, disrespectful, damaging, and unnecessary.

If the reason you fat-shame is that you "care" about the overweight individual's health, reevaluate your life choices. If you want to change the world and become a crusader for the obesity epidemic, get an education and become a nutritionist, wellness coach, or personal trainer. Don't be the douchebag yelling "Mooo!" out of the window of a moving car at the woman walking her dog. Pointing out that someone is fat does not encourage them to lose weight. It just doesn't work that way.

If you've never struggled with your weight, you wouldn't understand what it's like to be overweight. And that's okay; you're not expected to understand a situation that you've never had the opportunity to experience. But lack of experience does not equate to lack of empathy. Being overweight is hard. Obesity is not easy. And while on the outside looking in, it might look like a choice, it's more than that. It's an ingrained way of thinking, acting, and behaving that has resulted in severe health implications. And behavior that is so ingrained, habituated, and fed by addictive substances (sugar) is not something that goes away in a day. It won't go away with a heart-to-heart conversation. It will take time, intentional habit-reforming actions, and a dedication to learn what a healthy life looks like. So please keep that in mind if you want to "help" individuals completely transform their lives. It will take time. They are climbing a mountain, not walking up a flight of stairs.

While I am a passionate fitness instructor, with borderline too much energy and enthusiasm, I will not scream the weight off of you. And sometimes I see trainers do that. Their approach is that if you want to lose weight, you will work until you're on the brink of breaking and then push a little more. I get their intentions; they want you to work hard. But please, there is more to weight loss than exhausting exercise. When I think back on the days I had my personal trainer, while I hated the gym and the workouts, I remember I loved Jessica. She had compassion for her clients although she was not overweight herself, or had ever experienced being overweight. She knew what it meant to push someone out of their comfort zone. She understood that it was hard for me and could relate to me on that level. As a person new to fitness and exercise, that was huge for me: a trainer who understood that what she was putting me through was challenging, not a trainer who crushed my nonexistent exercise soul and killed any passion that might form because she was a drill sergeant with zero understanding of the daily struggles of being overweight. So for my trainers out there, have a heart and the passion to help people make healthier choices as they make their way up Mt. Weight Loss. Remember, they are on a long journey for lasting health, not a sprint back to "normal life."

Body-shaming is not something that you will experience only when overweight. I have experienced just as much negative unwanted and unwarranted opinions of my healthy weight as I did when I was overweight. Again, to the body-shamers, this treatment does not elicit change or action on my part. When I reached my healthy weight range and people started asking me if I did cocaine, that did not prompt me to give up my healthy lifestyle. When random men would comment on my pictures and say that I looked better with "meat on my bones," that did not deplete my drive to work out. When people post my pictures on social media and comment on how "gross" my hip bones are, that does not stop me from wanting to be healthy. And as a side note, I can't target my hip bones at the gym. I have wide, high-set, and prominent hip bones. There is no exercise that will decrease the shape of my hip bones. Commenting on and judging people's bodies do not produce anything positive. And doing so says more about the person making the comments than it does about the recipient. The point I am trying to drive home is to keep your body comments to yourself. If you can't say anything nice, don't say anything at all.

And for those who have received relentless comments from the body-shamers and the body police, you are not defined by other people's comments. You are more than what random, uneducated, and hurtful people say you are. Don't for one second let the opinion of a random stranger, online troll, or negative individual in your life make you think less of yourself. Always shine bright, dream big, and choose to be happy. There will always be people who want to bring you down in an attempt to pull themselves up. You're a lion in a world full of sheep. You're stronger than they will ever be. Remember that.

Stretch Marks: What do I think about them? Well, I have them, and they're not a big deal. My stretch marks faded as I lost weight. They are now a pale white color, and when I get a nice spray tan they are hardly noticeable. But they are not the end of the world, and they don't make me think less of myself! You can't control your stretch marks, so why waste energy on them? Focus on what you *can* control. Focus on creating a healthy life you will enjoy. Stretch marks don't mean anything. Skinny people have them. Boys have them. Fit girls have them. Whether you're small, tall, wide, or narrow, stretch marks do not discriminate! When you feel confident about yourself, who is going to notice the little lines on your body? Don't feel obligated to devalue yourself because someone else has a negative view of you. You can't change stretch marks. Either you have them or you don't.

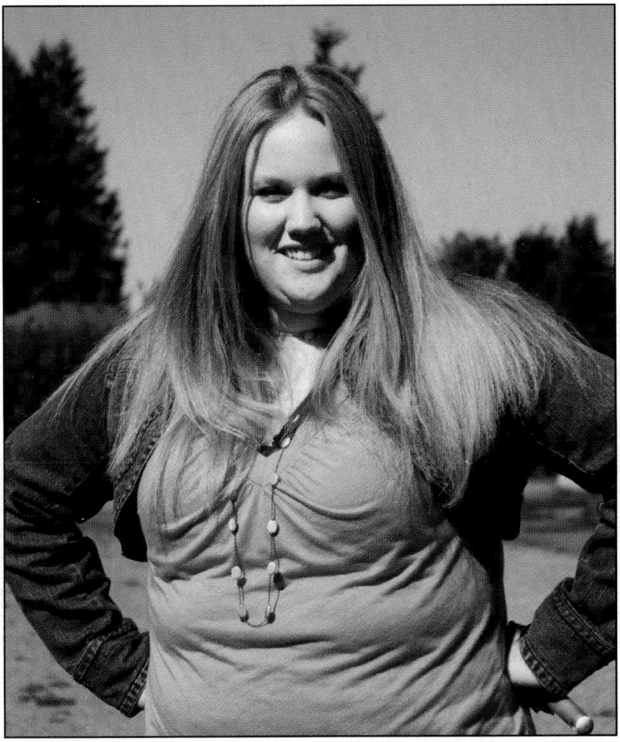

My high school senior year photos. During this photoshoot, I felt so uncomfortable in my own skin. This was the part in my journey where I thought I had already hit rock bottom . . . but had yet to see my highest weight on the scale. My wake-up call was slowly approaching.

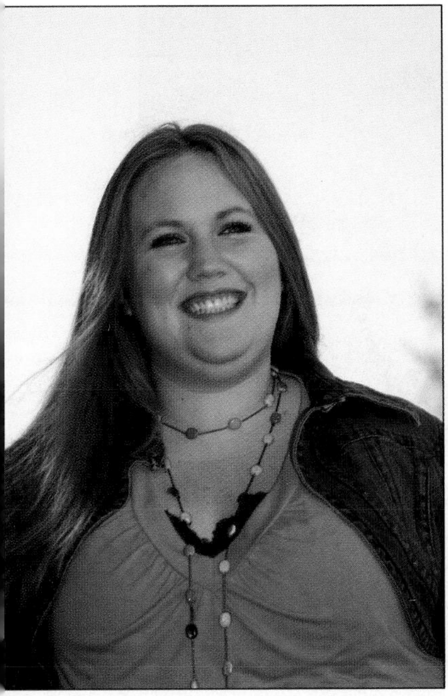

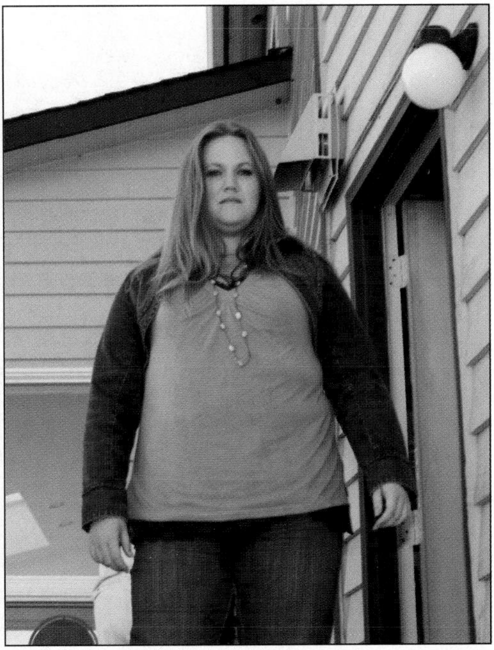

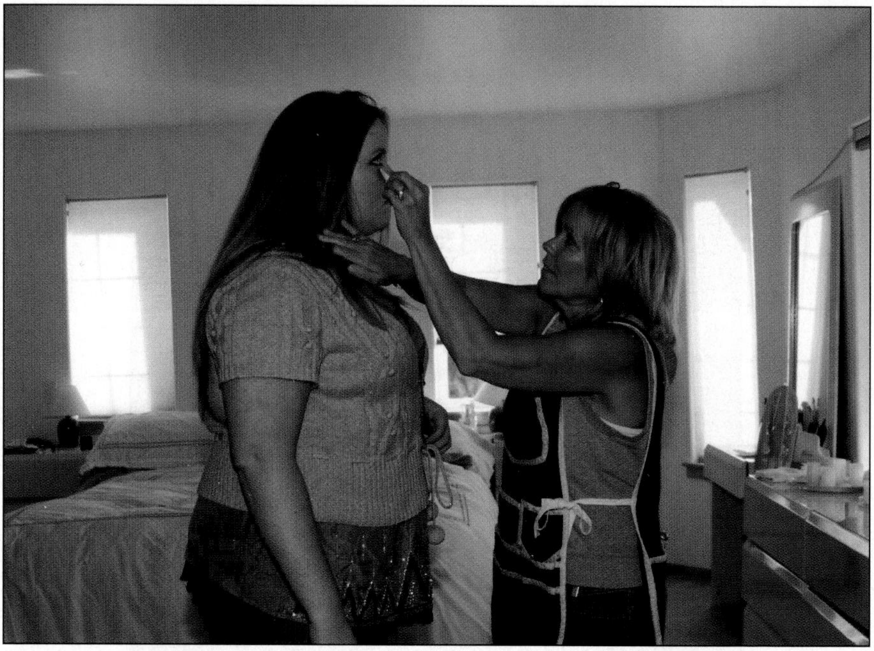

My mom doing my makeup in preparation for my high school senior photo.

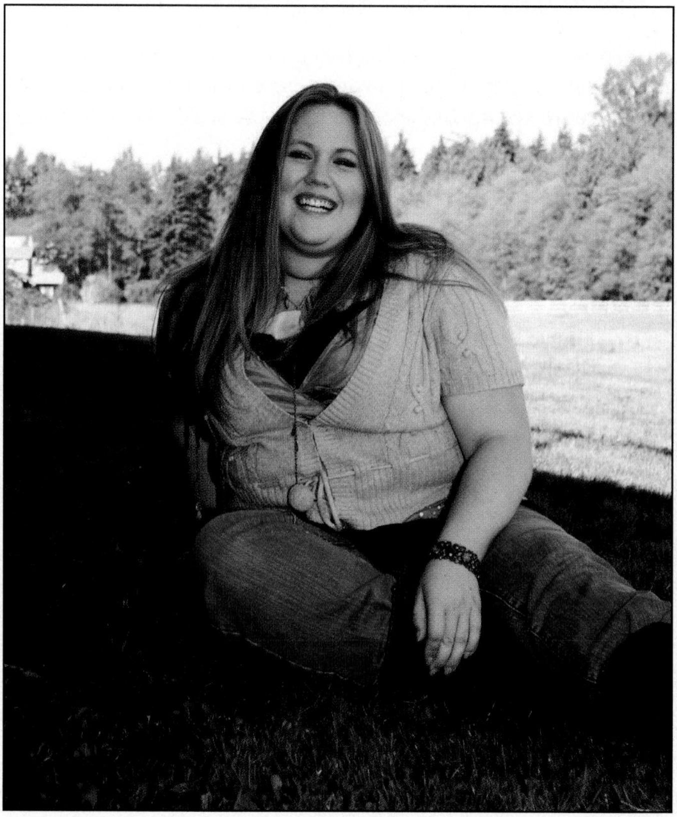

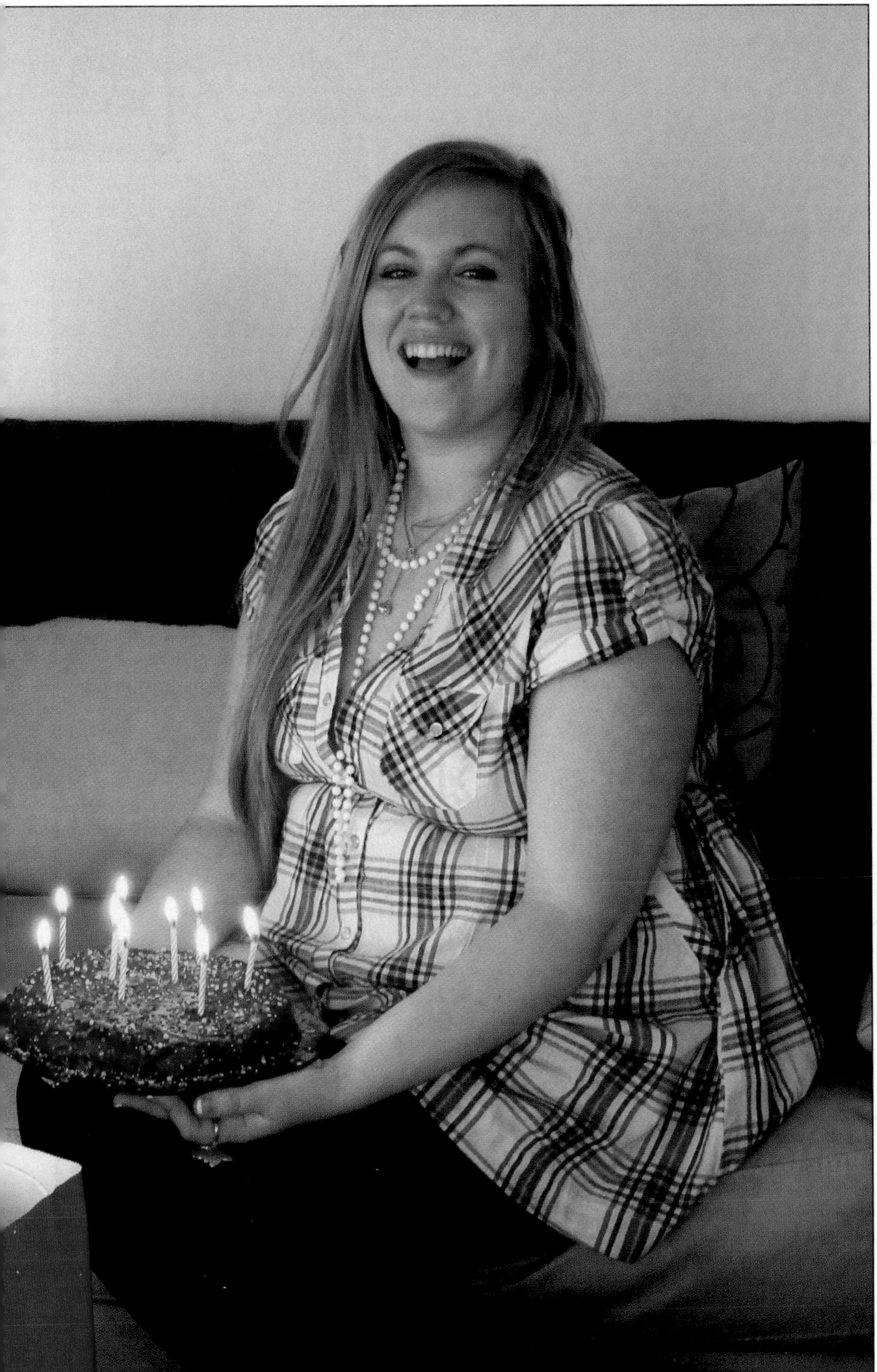

:elebrating my 21st birthday with my family. I was around 220 pounds when this picture vas taken. I had been vegan for almost two years but I was still in the junk-food vegan :tage. This was my first attempt at making a vegan cake.

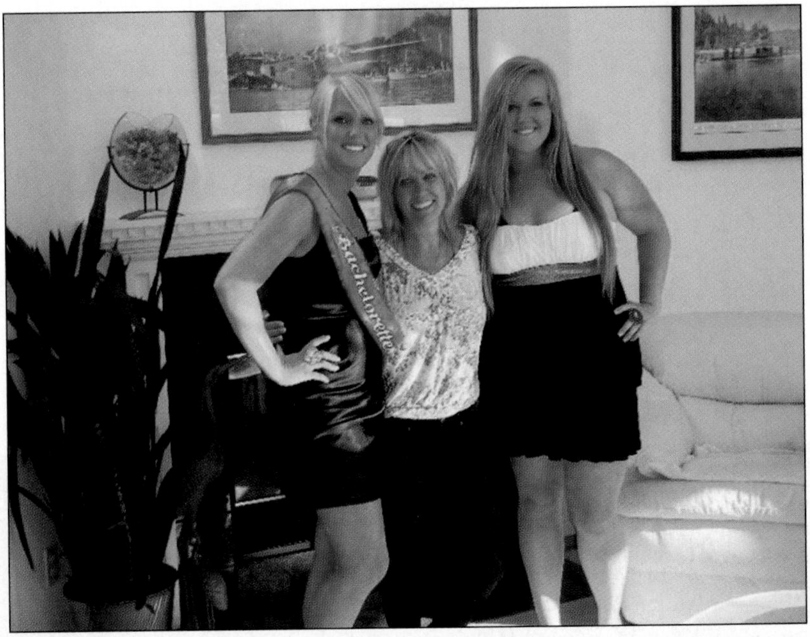

Left to right: my sister Ganelle, my mom, and me. My sister and I were on our way out for Ganelle's bachelorette party. This picture was taken a few months after my 21st birthday. My sister does and always has resembled a Barbie doll; I was envious of her in that black dress.

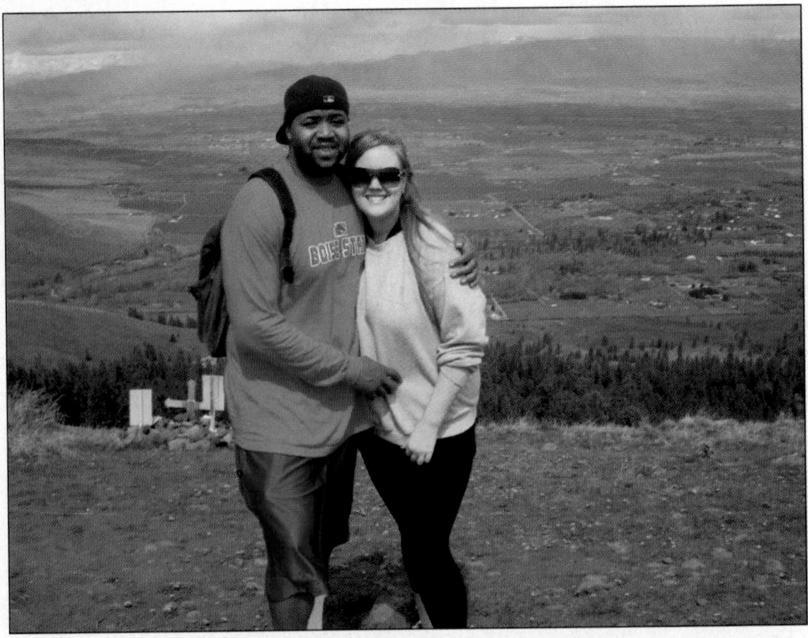

Dre and I hiking Manastash Ridge in Ellensburg, Washington. I was never one for hikes until I met Dre—we routinely hiked this trail. This picture was taken a few months after we started dating. I was around 230 pounds when we first met. Fast forward 3 years, he proposed to me on the same hiking trail.

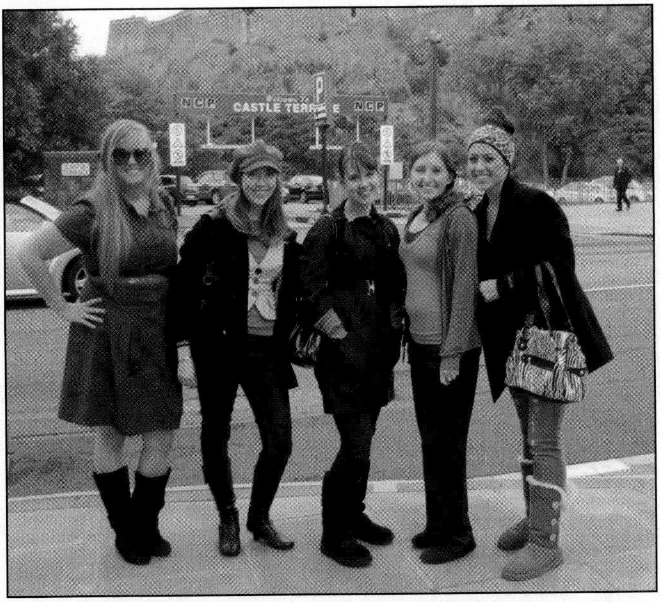

First day in Edinburgh, Scotland, walking around the city with my new flatmates. I was around 220 pounds in this picture. From left to right: me, Clarissa, Megan, Jessica, and Kristin.

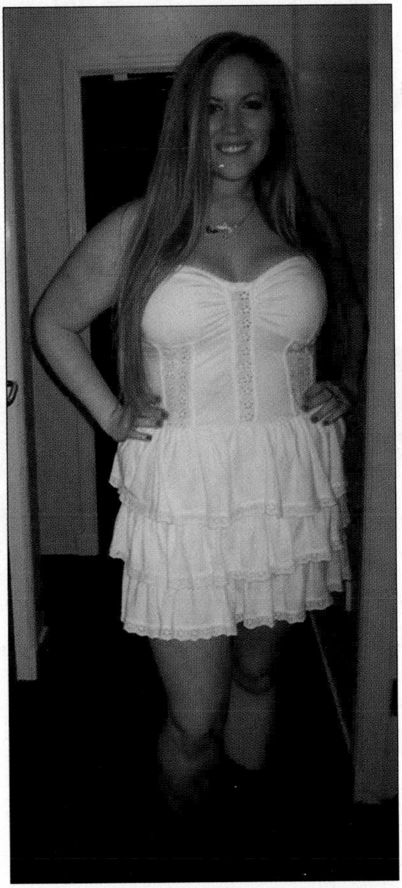

Ready for a night out in Edinburgh, Scotland. This was taken shortly before I came home for the holidays over winter break. I was around 190 pounds and I felt amazing. I did not know how much I weighed (I didn't have access to a scale while abroad) but I knew that I was losing weight and I felt great. Not having access to vegan junk food and walking everywhere was paying off!

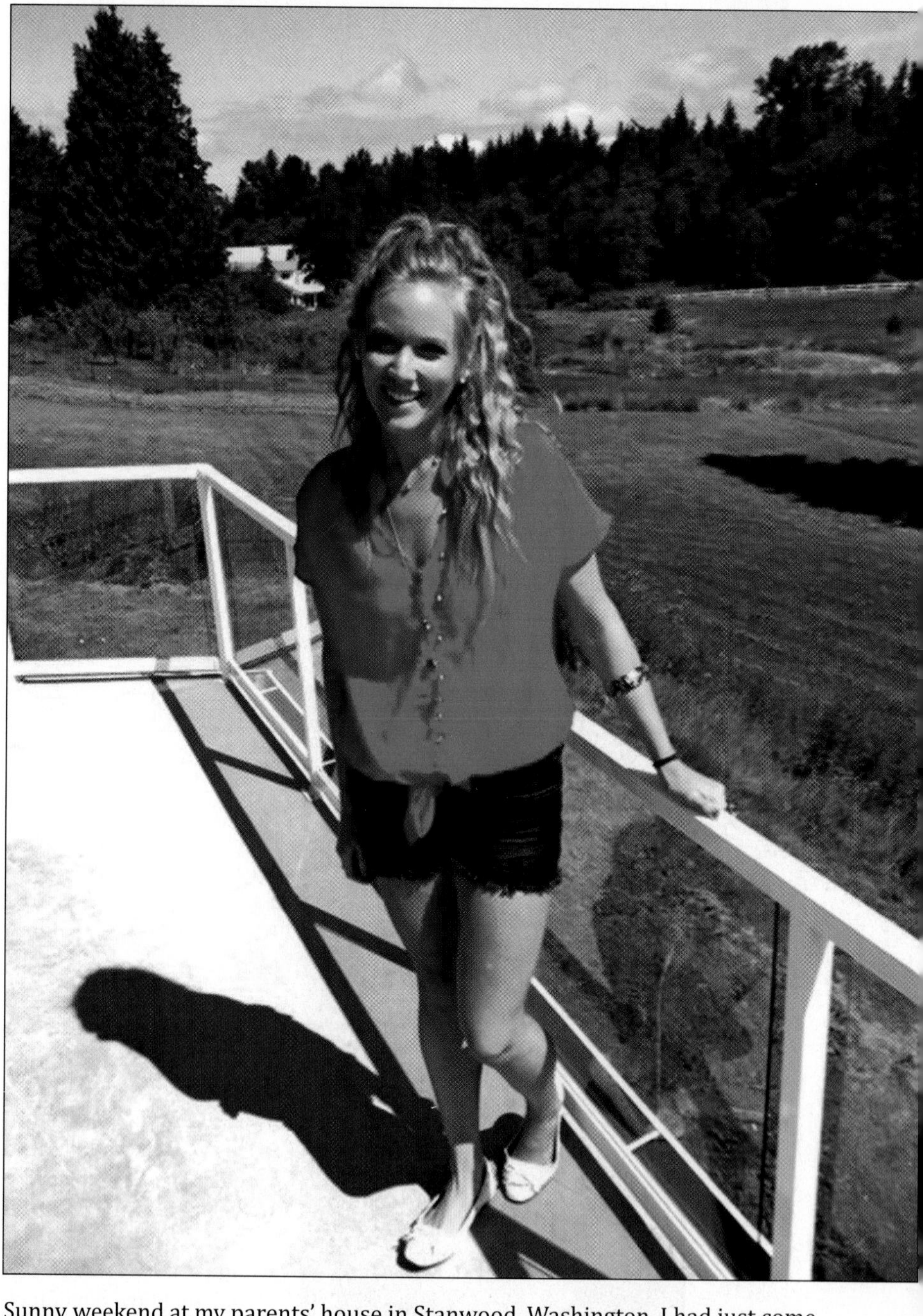

Sunny weekend at my parents' house in Stanwood, Washington. I had just come downstairs and Dre said "you look so pretty, we need to take pictures!" I was around 150 pounds in this picture and feeling like a million bucks.

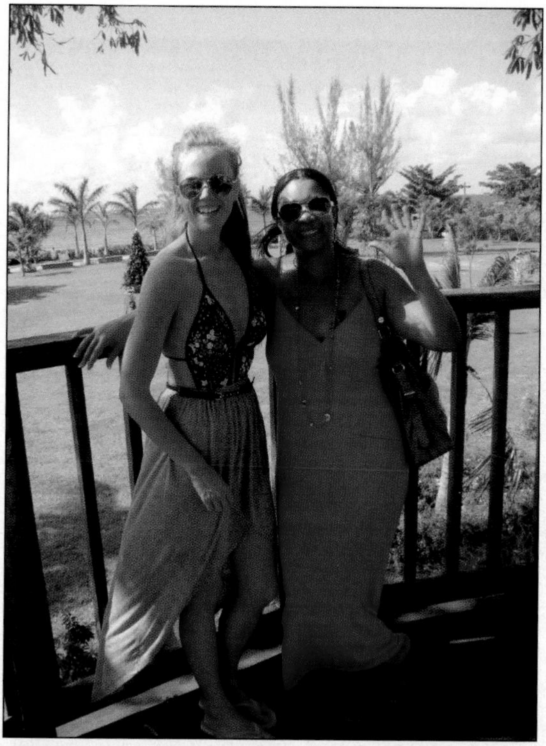

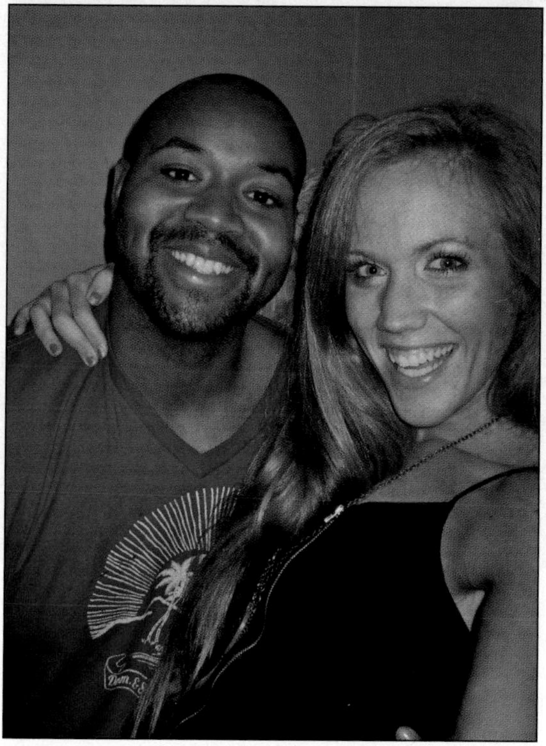

Montego Bay, Jamaica, on a trip to meet my new family. Dre grew-up in Jamaica and moved to the United States with his mom in his early teens. Shortly after we got engaged, he took me to Jamaica over Christmas to meet the rest of his family (I'm pictured in the top photo with his mom, my new mother-in law). I was around 140 pounds in this picture.

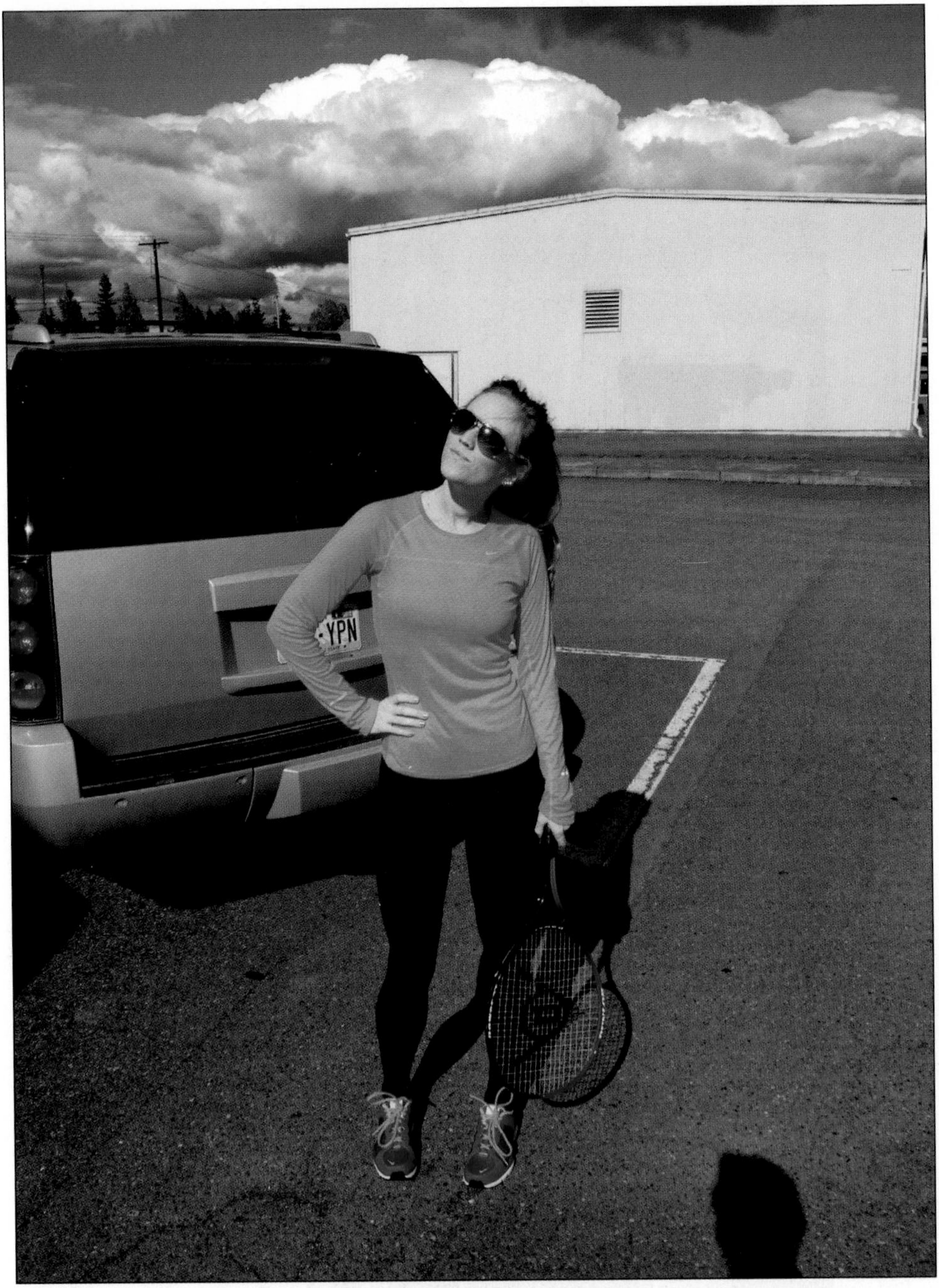

Although my tennis game has much to be desired, Dre and my family enjoy playing. I more so just tag along to be a body on the court for a game of doubles, but it's a fun way to get my heart rate up! This picture was taken 10 weeks after my tummy tuck; I was easing my way back into exercise and tennis was a good way to stay active without overdoing it.

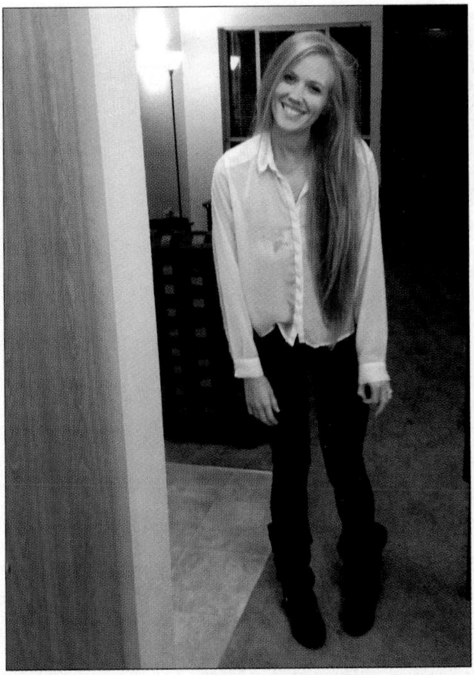

Dre likes jeans, but I've always been the "yoga-pants-are-real-pants" type. So anytime I wear jeans, Dre feels the need to document it. This was one of those times.

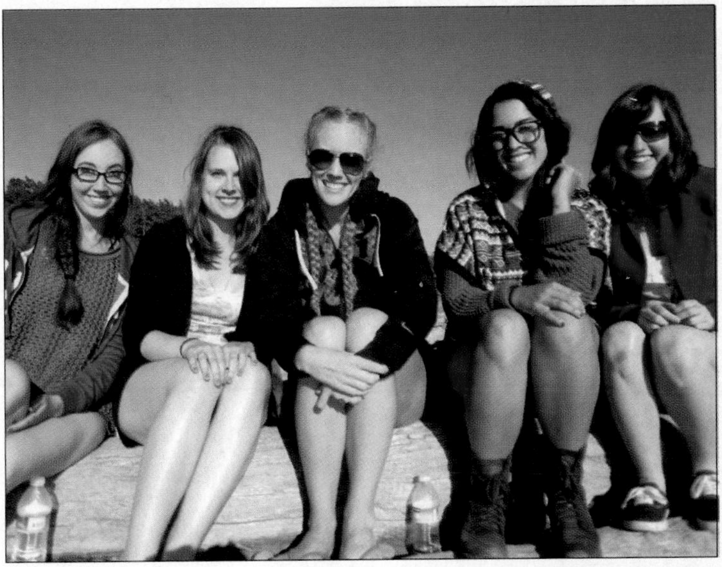

My roommates from my time abroad all flew to Seattle from various places of the world the week before my wedding. Our year in Scotland together created a bond for life. From left to right: Clarissa, Megan, me, Kristin, and Jessica.

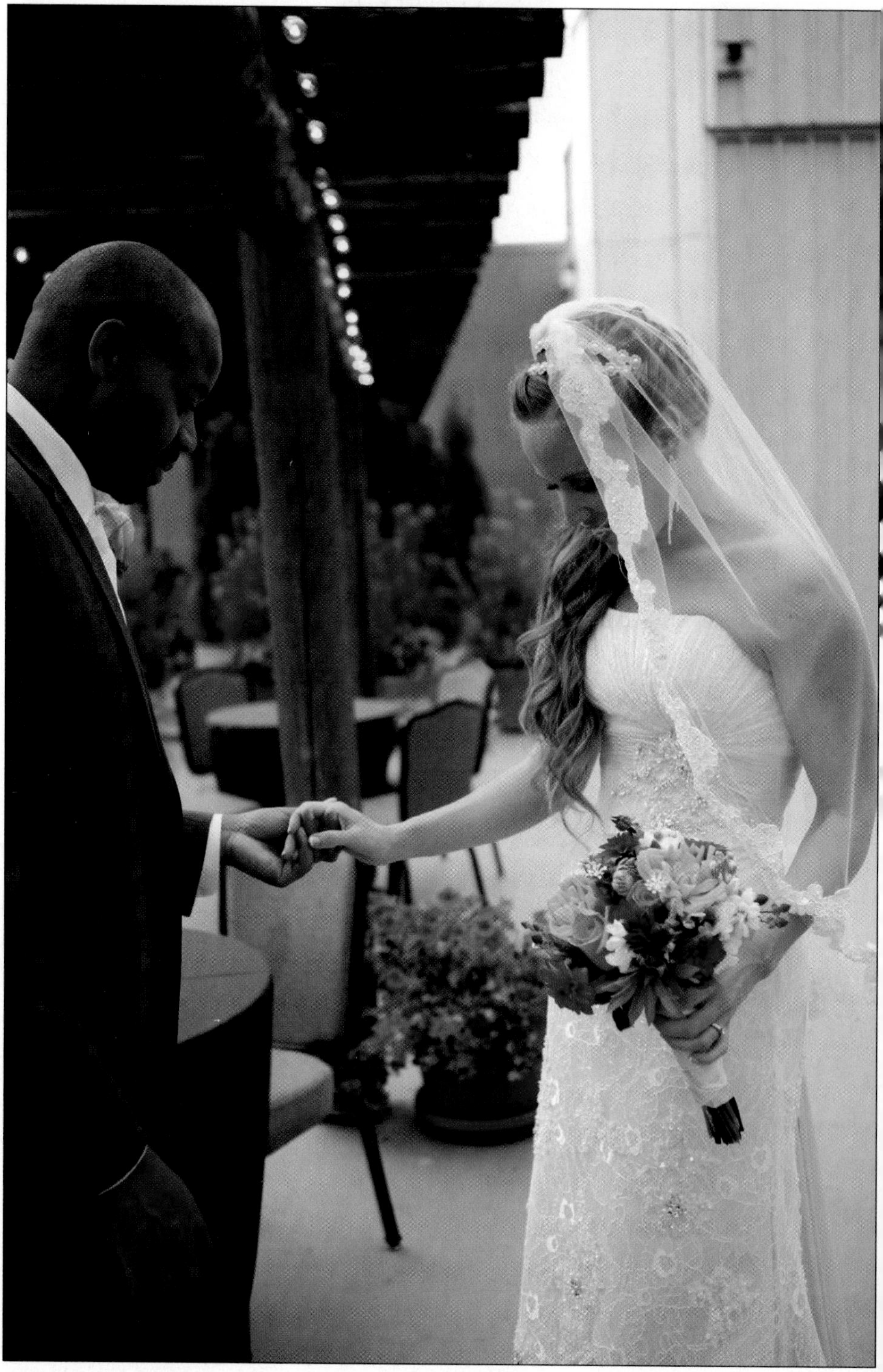

The day dreams are made of . . . marrying the love of my life, in the dress of my dreams.
(Photo Credit: Yuen Lui Studio)

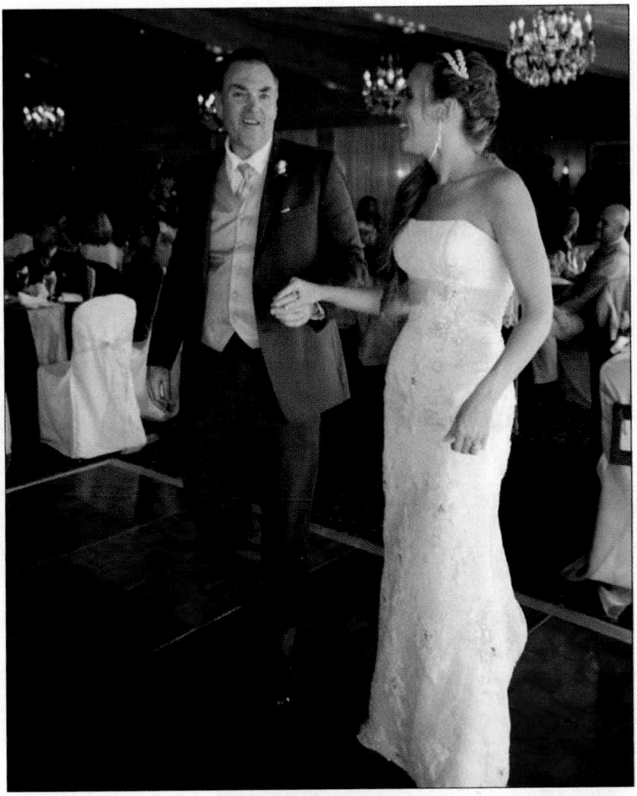

Father-daughter dance. (Photo Credit: Yuen Lui studio)

My amazing siblings and their spouses—from left to right: Madii, Bryce, Me, Dre, Ganelle, and Troy. My family stood by my side every step of my fitness journey.

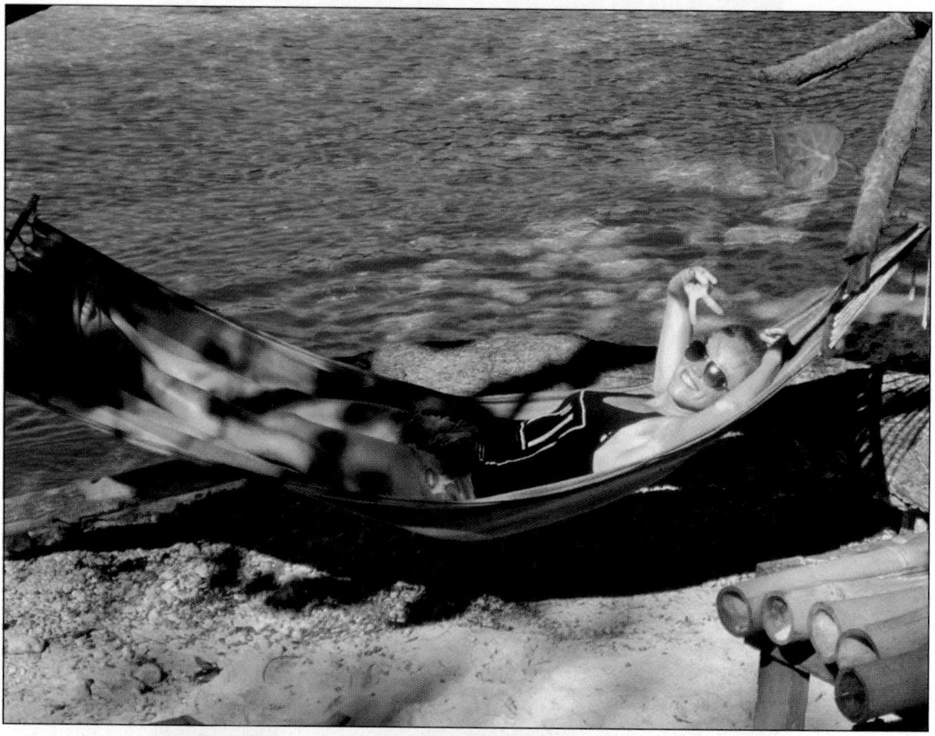

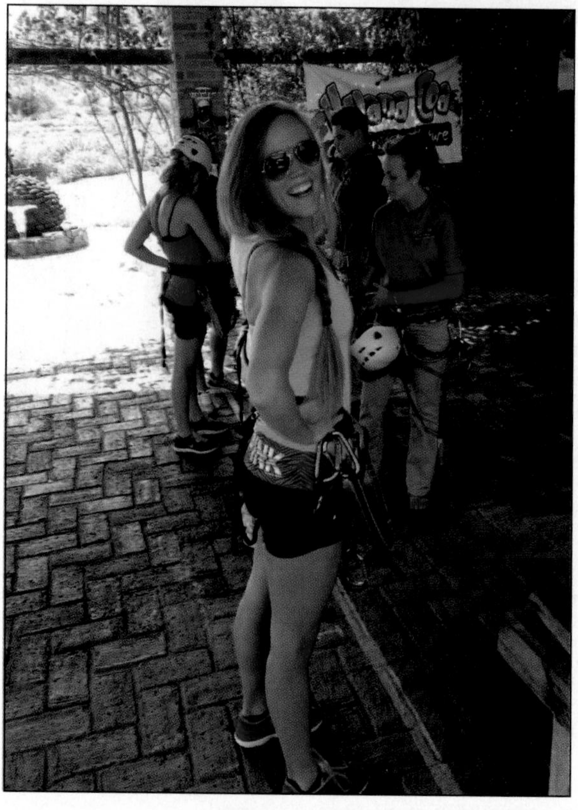

Honeymoon in Mazatlán, Mexico, ready to Zipline. Never in my wildest dreams would I have pictured myself flying through the air, with all my weight dependent on a rope! I felt amazing on my honeymoon. All my hard work had paid off. I was able to participate in activities that I had never dared to do before because I was fearful of my size and weight.

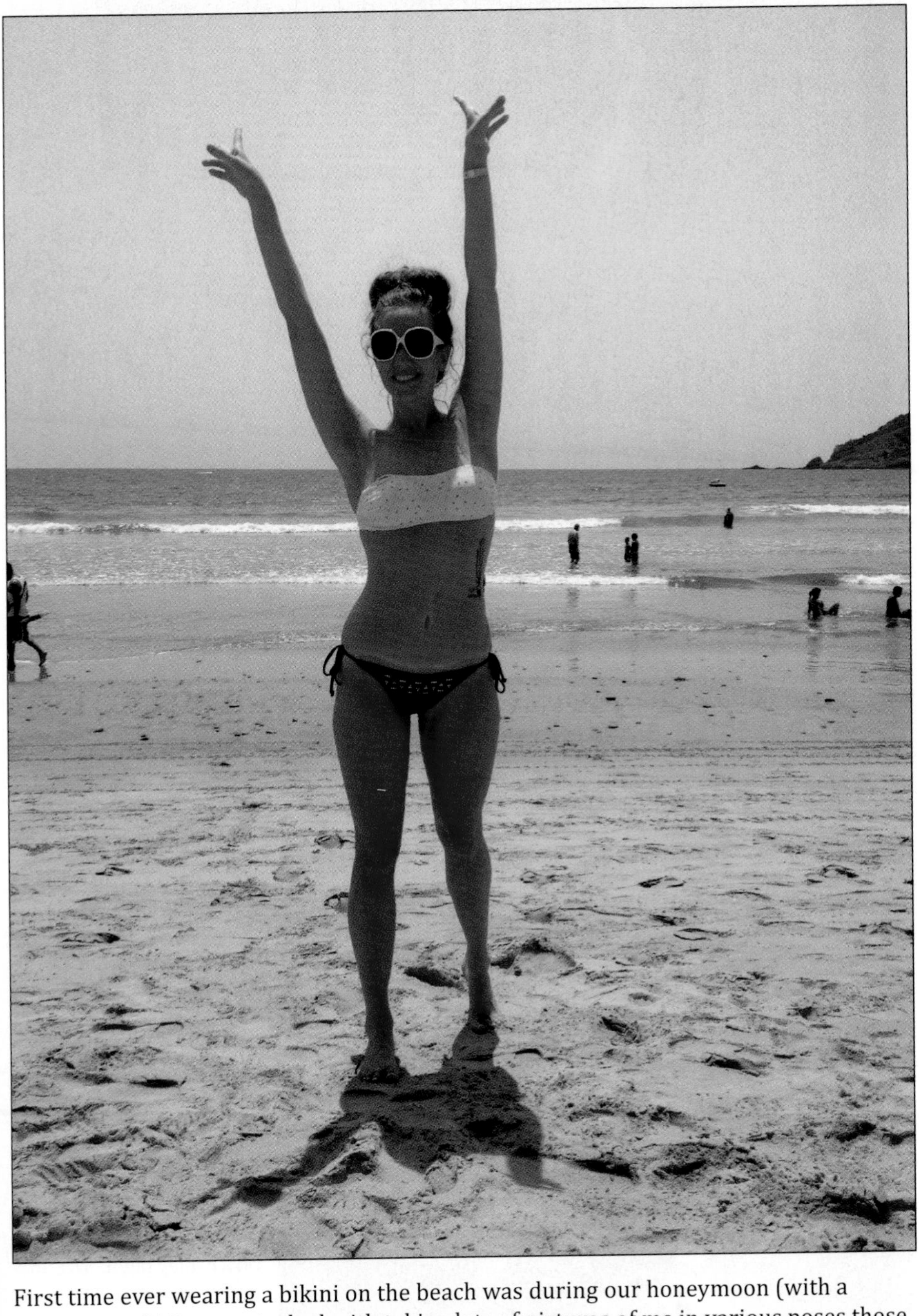

First time ever wearing a bikini on the beach was during our honeymoon (with a henna tattoo)! Dre was tasked with taking lots of pictures of me in various poses those couple of weeks. It was my dream to prance on the beach in an itty bitty bikini and I had finally accomplished it! That moment on the beach was one that I had day dreamed about for years.

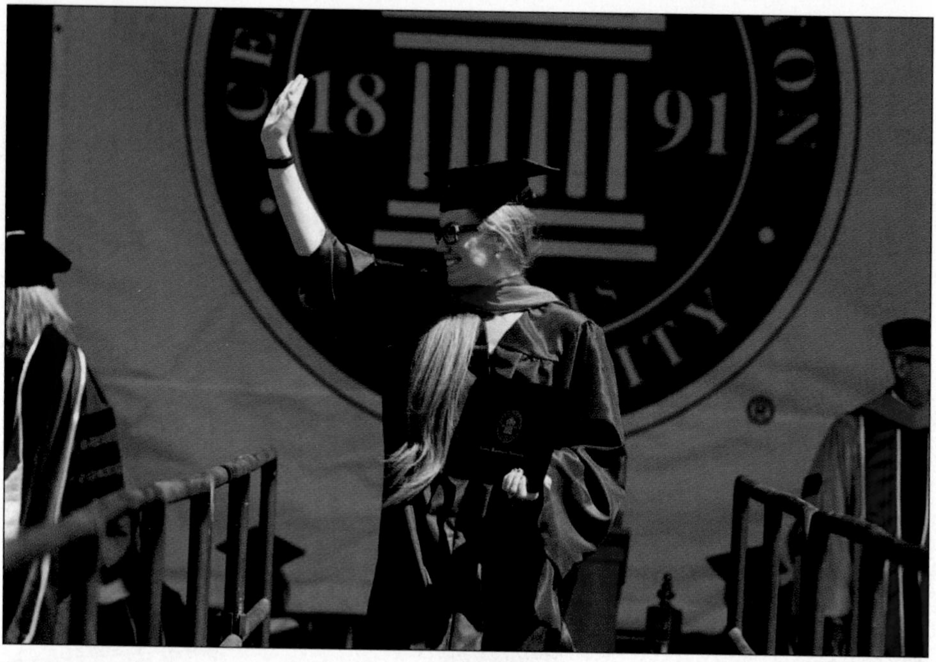

Graduating from Central Washington University with my Educational Specialist Degree in School Psychology. Graduate school is no easy task, and completing a three-year full-time master's degree program is most certainly not at the top of anyone's "most enjoyable things" list. I stuck to my fitness goals and my school goals . . . and came out successful. This was the weekend I decided to commit to training for a bikini competition—I check off one goal, and on to the next.

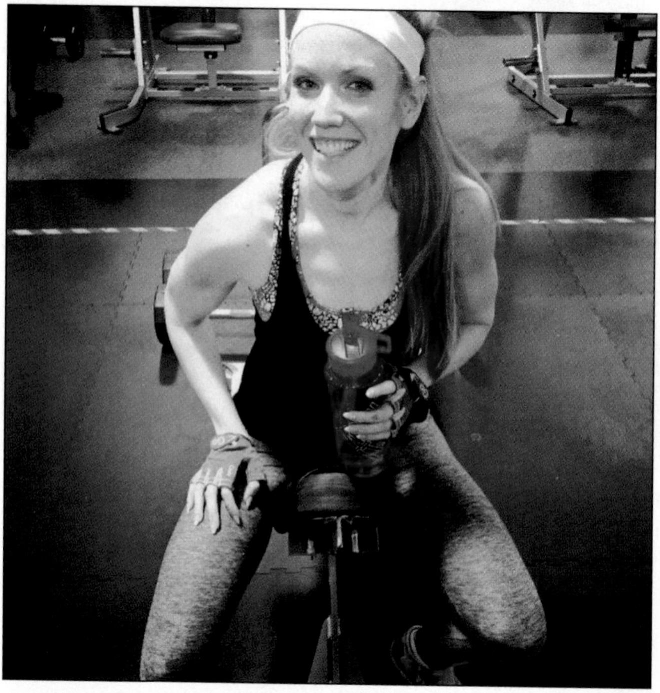

A few moments before this picture was taken, Dre looked and me and said "we are on vacation in San Jose, California . . . and we went to the gym on a Friday night." Dreams take dedication. This was a week before my first bikini competition. A goal that big takes a heavy dose of commitment. One that he and I were both ready and willing to make together.

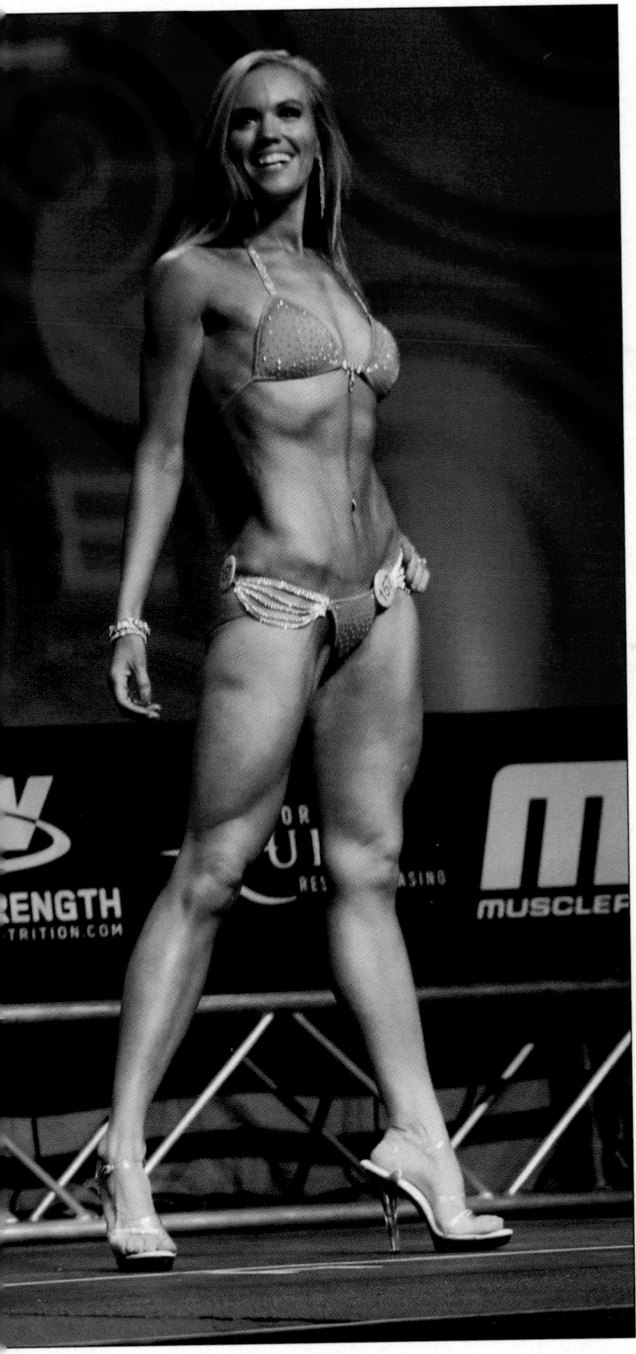

Bikini competitions are a division of body building, and training for them takes a whole new level of training and dedication. I prepared under the direct guidance and supervision of a coach who trains and conditions plant-fed competitors. The diet and training required to compete is not part of my regular regime. For me, it was about showing that I could accomplish anything I put my mind to—that a girl who once weighed 256 pounds could stand on stage with the best-of-the-best in a sparkly bikini. After I completed my first bikini competition, I was crushed that I did not place as well as I had hoped. Although it was my very first show, I had put so much dedication and commitment into my training, that I was left feeling defeated when I walked away with a low placing. It was my mom's encouraging words that reminded me of how far I had come and how much I have accomplished over the years; that I had worked too hard to be disappointed in myself. And as always, she was 100% right. I pushed through another few weeks of training and stepped on stage again. The second show was about me and my personal progress, not a trophy.
(Photo Credit: Mark Mason)

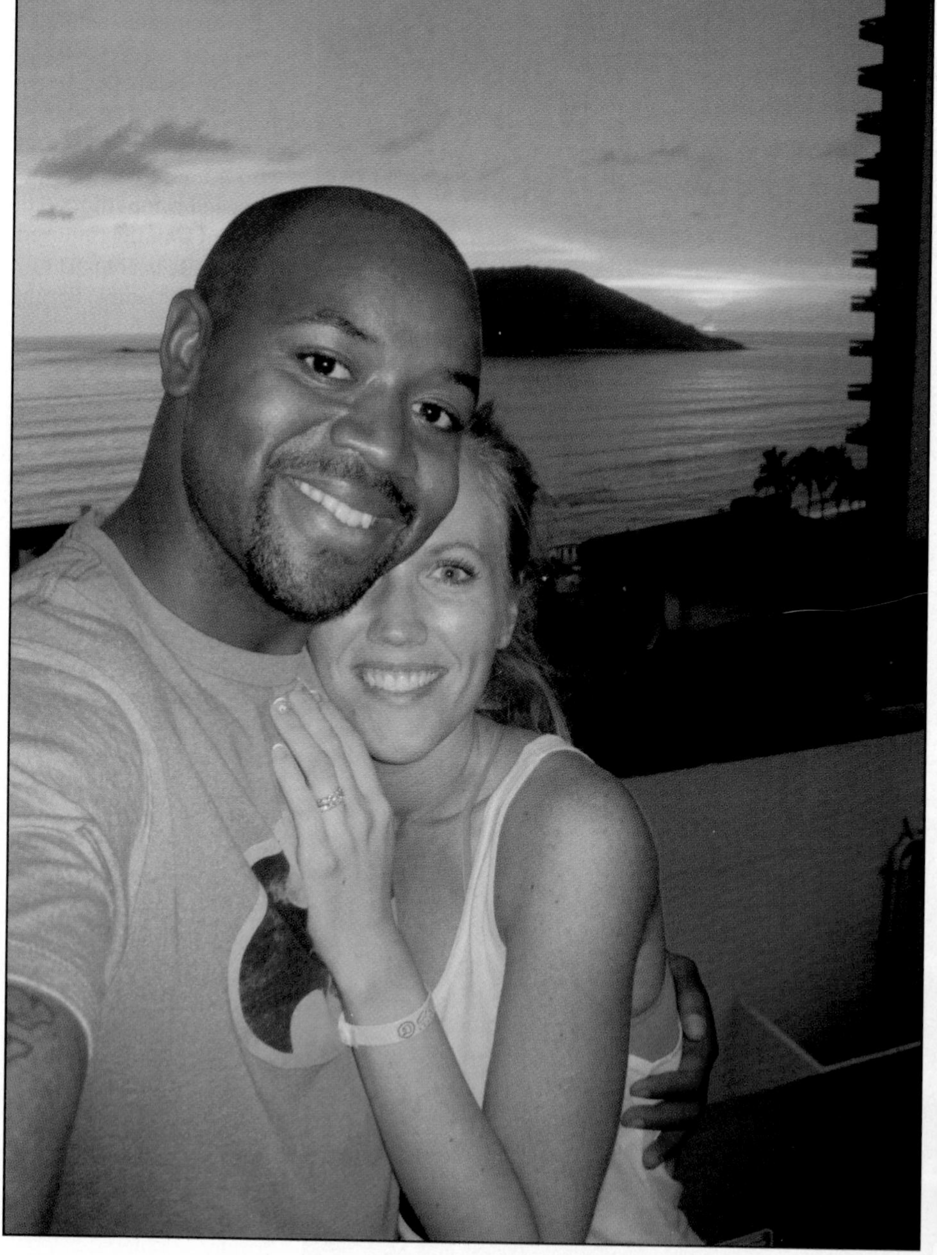

Happy and in love.

They might fade, but there are no magic lotions that will make them go away. So just accept them and move on.

I know some people spend mass amounts of time frantically worrying and stressing about their stretch marks. I know they are a big deal for some people and I don't want to minimize that. So I want you to know that I understand how frustrating stretch marks can be, but I also want to share that you don't have to stress about them. They are not something that will matter when your life is oozing with health and when you're radiating with positivity. They will always be there. They might fade, and they might not. But ultimately, it's important to accept them and then focus on something that you can control. You can rock whatever outfit you want with or without stretch marks. I wear a bikini with stretch marks, and I don't even think twice! It's not worth stressing over because I can't change them.

Changed Body Image: You've spent your entire journey focusing on losing weight, and now the person in the mirror does not reflect the person you knew your whole life. Or you lose all this weight, reach your goal weight, and still feel overweight. Both are completely normal and expected experiences. I've experienced both of them. When people refer to me as "skinny" or "small," I'm shocked! I look around to see whom they are talking about! I spent the majority of my life overweight. Small is new and something that I am *still* learning to adjust to. While my weight is no longer constantly on my mind, I find myself more sensitive to weight-related comments. I also feel that I focus on clothing sizes more than the typical person. But it makes sense, and I'm not crazy. And if you're facing similar scenarios, you're not crazy either! My entire life I was hypersensitive about my weight. And that hypersensitivity does not simply go away as the scale changes. Your mental schemas don't shift as you lose weight. There is no established automatic process between shrinking body weight and new and improved body image.

When you're overweight, you know it. It's permanently on your mind. You walk in a room and instantly scan it to see if you're the largest person there. If you have to share a seat close to someone, you wonder if you can fit there comfortably, or if they will worry about the amount of space you will take when you sit next to them. When you're waiting to approach a ride at an amusement park, will you be able to fit in the ride? Will the seat belt buckle? Do you exceed the weight limit? If you forget a jacket when you're going out, you can't simply borrow just anybody's jacket if you get cold. You wear extended sizes that the majority of your friends don't even know exist. You can't throw on your BFF's shorts if you forgot to pack pajama bottoms. You have an irrational fear of sitting on something and having it break. You question the bench at the park or the swings. Will they be able to support your weight? You daydream of cuddling on your significant other's lap without feeling like you're smothering or crushing them. Your weight is relentlessly on your mind. And that does not go away simply because you reached your goal weight.

It's an adjustment and it takes time and practice to accept the new you. I don't have a magic method for teaching you how to accept the new you and realize your new weight. This is something that will come with time and continued healthy living. Eventually, your healthy habits will become second nature and your life will reflect all the positive changes you worked so hard to make. The person in the mirror will become more familiar and you will learn to embrace them.

But let's talk about body dysmorphia. Body dysmorphia is a real thing. Essentially, it's a mental illness that distorts a person's perception of their body. Individuals become hyperfocused on their "imperfections" and controlled by a twisted and distorted view of themselves. Sometimes it's a specific facial feature such as the nose or ears, whereas other times the distortion is related to weight or size. Does everyone who loses weight have body dysmorphia? No. But keep in mind that mental illnesses are on a spectrum. There is a typical end and a disordered end. *Everyone* is on the same spectrum, but when your brain swings too far toward the disordered end, *then* you see those with mental illnesses and severe symptoms. But the everyday average person can experience some symptoms of various mental illnesses without having mental illness. It's a spectrum. This is why you can have disordered eating habits without having an eating disorder.

You can be compulsive and picky about cleanliness and order without having obsessive-compulsive disorder. The closer you fall toward the disordered end, the more symptoms you will exhibit and experience.

Can the everyday average person experience symptoms of body dysmorphia? Absolutely. Does the everyday average person have body dysmorphia? No. It's not a common mental illness. While I do have a background and degree in psychology, my scope of practice is school psychology. I do psychoeducational (psychology plus education/learning) evaluations for special education eligibility. I conduct evaluations that recognize when disorders are present, but I do not diagnose mental health disorders or prescribe medication. I identify disabilities that are impacting a student's ability to learn and progress in a general education setting. Then I work with a team of teachers, counselors, and specialists as well as the parents to help develop an appropriate educational plan and path that will meet the student's individual needs. Sounds pretty fancy, huh? My background is not mental health based or focused. But what my background in psychology does help me to understand is that our brains are complex, and that "normal" has a widespread range with a lot of variation.

I was overweight my entire teenage life and through my early twenties. I have no memory of ever being below two hundred pounds. I began lying about my weight in the seventh grade. While I lost weight over the course of five years, I rapidly experienced a huge shift in size and weight toward the end of my journey (when I critically evaluated my E.F.F.O.R.T.). That change and drop in weight, size, and scale readings came quickly. And my brain did not have time to adapt to the "new" me. I would look in the mirror and see a smaller person . . . but I had been so focused on losing weight for so long that part of me felt incomplete unless I was chasing a number on the scale. I wasn't unhealthy, and I have always maintained a healthy weight for my height. But I had a difficult time adjusting to reaching the top of Mt. Weight Loss. I still felt big even though I was small—because I was overweight for so long. I still reached for large and extra-large sizes when shopping. Eventually, I had to have Dre pick all my clothes for me because I would pick clothes that I drowned in! Your brain has a mental image of you, your self-reflection. It will take time for your brain to adjust to a new reflection.

When you're experiencing this adjusting reflection process, it can be depressing. You can begin to think, "Why did I lose all this weight if I'm still unhappy with how I look?" I get it. I've been there! But just know that *this* is part of your journey too: the mental aspect of weight loss, the mental acceptance of reaching a healthy weight range and shifting to the maintenance track versus the weight-loss climb. The ability to accept the new person you see in the mirror does not happen overnight. Your reflection was of a different person for so long, so it can feel strange to see a new person in the mirror or in pictures. It can also be hard to accept the progress you are making. You might begin to pick small imperfections and catastrophize them because you're so used to working toward a physical goal. Your new reflection is treated like a stranger because you don't really have a relationship with the person you see in the mirror. It might sound odd, but it happens. And if you're experiencing this right now, it's normal! I promise.

So what can you do? Practice self-love and positive self-talk. Take time to appreciate how far you have come and all your hard work. I was so focused on losing weight that occasionally I lost track of all the things I had accomplished along the way. Don't lose sight of the real goal, a healthy and happy life. If you're having a difficult time accepting whom you see in the mirror, whether it be because of loose skin, stretch marks, an unfamiliar reflection, etc., take a mental step back and reflect on all that you have accomplished. Reflect on the dedication that it took to get you where you are today. The hours you spent working out, the effort you put into replacing unhealthy eating habits with healthy ones, the times you turned down mouthwatering cake—all those accomplishments add up to the person you see in the mirror! And that person deserves your love, respect, and appreciation. I would not be the person I am today without the 256-pound Sharee busting her butt and staying focused on her goals. I am not ashamed of who I was, because she made me who I am today.

So take time to appreciate the new person in the mirror, the person whom you created by staying dedicated to your goals, consistent with your healthy eating, and determined to replace those unhealthy eating habits with healthy ones. The person you see in the mirror was forged with blood, sweat, tears, and self-determination. The fact that you reached your goal is a miracle. Sadly, many people give up halfway up the climb. The conditions of the climb are just too much for them and they either turn back, give up, or sit down and make camp. And they continue to live a good portion of their life halfway to their goals. But not you—you made it! You beat the odds and completely changed your life! Think about how incredible that is. Be proud. And it might seem easy to downplay your accomplishment, because it's only weight loss—but trust me, what you did and what you're doing right now are amazing and worth celebrating on a daily basis.

The "You've Gone Too Far" Crowd: So maybe you're not at this place on your journey yet, but give it some time, and those people will arrive. The people who say things like, "You're too thin," "Geez, you look anorexic now," "Don't you ever eat?" or "You looked better before." Those people will find you and they will try to bring you down. And they can be successful if you let them. I remember the first time I experienced this. I was approached by an online magazine to share my story and I was so excited! I spent hours detailing my interview answers and ensuring that I conveyed a message that would help inspire others.

The day the article posted, while there was positive feedback, I received a lot of "She's too thin," "She looked better with meat on her bones," "I bet she has an eating disorder," "She looks like a walking skeleton of skin," and "She doesn't look like a woman anymore." The comments were hurtful and from complete strangers. I spent hours detailing the healthy way I lost weight and reached my goals, and all these people could do was focus on how they didn't like how I looked anymore. Their definition of beauty and what they found attractive were more important than my health. Initially, I was devastated and the experience made me not want to share my story online anymore. How could complete strangers make such hurtful comments about another person with whom they had no personal relationship? I was shocked and upset.

I could have justified deleting my blog after that article was posted. I could have continued my journey and just shared it with my friends and family. But I didn't. I decided in that moment that I wouldn't care what random people would have to say about me. What they might say about me would say more about them than me. Why should I care if some random person finds me more attractive when I was bigger? Why should I care if some person behind a computer screen thinks I look too thin? I don't care, and you don't have to care either!

With the growth of my blog came the influx of hate mail and online trolls. Unfortunately, if you allow people to send anonymous questions out of respect for individual privacy, you will often have people who abuse that privilege, such as individuals who sit behind a screen and send hateful messages in an attempt to derail you and your mission to spread hope for healthy weight-loss methods. Again, you can choose to react—or you can choose to piss people off with kindness.

I have never responded to a hateful or hurtful message. I delete it and move on. But the person who sent me the message has to return to my blog daily to see if I have responded . . . and I never do. So they continue to be bombarded with positivity and healthiness even in the midst of their hate. I prefer to allow people to drown in their own hate-filled puddle rather than splash around in it with them. And the older I get, the more I understand that not every situation needs a reaction. It's okay to not respond. It's okay to simply ignore people who can't carry themselves in a respectful, appropriate way. Do I think I am higher or above them? No, absolutely not. I simply don't need to entertain people who lack common respect for and decency toward others. I choose my interactions wisely. Because they do and will shape you.

So you can ignore the individuals online, but what about the people in real life who want to devalue your hard work? The friends or family members who constantly tell you that you're too thin or have gone too far? Well, sometimes you might go overboard, and your family is right. It's easy to do when you're so focused on losing weight. It can be hard to not want to keep pushing the boundaries of the scale. The steep hike up Mt. Weight Loss is adrenaline pumping. You get the rush from seeing the numbers drop on the scale. An effort to create a healthy life can turn into an addiction to weight loss. So consult with your doctor and establish a healthy weight range for you. That way, when people want to argue with you about your weight, you will know that you're healthy. It will help you to mentally stay strong when negative people are trying to bring you down.

If you are within a healthy weight range, and individuals continue to try insulting your hard work, you can either bring to their attention that their behavior will not be tolerated or choose to ignore it. A simple "I worked hard to get here and I'm very happy with my progress" is oftentimes enough to stop someone from talking. But every once in a while you will get an individual who just can't take the hint. That's when you can politely but firmly tell them that your weight is none of their business. Your happiness means more to you than their opinion of what you should weigh or look like. Sometimes you have to be straightforward with individuals; don't always assume that everyone has excellent social-pragmatic skills. As someone who assesses people daily for social-skill deficits, I can tell you that it's more common than you think.

"Real women have curves." That comment really annoys me. The people who choose to use that comment don't seem to understand how the human body works. You don't get to pick where your curves go. You don't get to decide how much like an hourglass your body shape is. By the way, I did not have curves when I was overweight; I had rolls. Here's some more knowledge for you, in case you're in the back and need some reminding: womanhood is not measured by your waist-to-hip ratio. I was gorgeous when I was overweight and I am gorgeous now. You are gorgeous right now in this moment, and that will not change.

Food Is "Love" Club Members: You may come from a family that does not support your weight loss. It is not your fault whether they feel a sense of inadequacy or that your healthy choices force them to reflect on their own unhealthy food choices. Sadly, I've seen it happen both with my friends and with individuals who share their stories with me. They work so hard to reach their goals, yet their families seemingly go out of their way to drag them down, constantly implying that the person losing weight has an eating disorder because they no longer want to eat fast food, or purchasing bad foods in an attempt to sabotage the individual's progress. It's sad, but it happens.

Some families show their love through food. We all have that one person in our family who is genuinely offended if you refuse to eat their homemade treats. I get it! Are they intentionally trying to sabotage your goals? No. But can you risk eating something that might put you on a slippery slope and have you sneaking into the kitchen late at night to eat more? No! Because remember, moderation does not work for everyone. And oftentimes, just that "one bite" is all it takes to send you into an unplanned treat season that turns into a full-on, overindulgent eating spree.

So talk to the family member whose heart breaks every time you turn down their homemade goodies. Give them the whole "It's not you, it's me" talk. I have had people argue with me about trying something they baked even though it's not vegan. I state, "No, thank you, but it looks delicious," and they continue to try to convince me to eat it. It's annoying, but I don't get angry. I simply continue to say no thank you and then excuse myself from the conversation or situation.

If food is the love language of your family, contribute something healthy to family gatherings or share a recipe with the best cook and ask if it's something they would like to make. Tell the pushy family member that while you would love to indulge in their triple-chocolate cheesecake, right now you have to take a rain check—but you would love to try their cranberry salad! Or ask if they know any yummy recipes you could try that would mesh with your goals. People who speak food love recipes! So even if you can't eat their signature dish, at least they can still share something with you. Remember, their language is food. So this will help them be able to speak to you in the best way they know how.

On the other hand, maybe this scenario is all too familiar: you have family members who intentionally try to sabotage your goals. Their reasoning might be driven by pure selfishness, or it could be that they don't understand anything other than food language. Either way, it's stressful and difficult to face on a continual basis.

Some people have family members who do not share food out of love. They intentionally attempt to sabotage your goals. And unfortunately, family is difficult to break up with, especially if you live under the same roof. So how do you tackle that issue? First, talk to the family members directly. Tell them what you're feeling and what you're seeing. They might not admit that they are being intentional in attempting to hold you back from your goals, but they might see the impact that it has on you and respect your requests.

If they insist on buying your "favorite" foods because they love you, post on the refrigerator a new list of favorite foods. Sometimes they might not know what to buy for you, so they stick to what they do know. You see this as sabotage and they see you as being ungrateful. So to help reduce conflict, make a specific list of foods you would love if they randomly purchased for you: grapes, apples, bananas, mixed nuts, etc. This list will help your family when shopping and will also help you feel more prepared for whatever arrives in the kitchen.

It can also be helpful to keep your food in separate places. On those days when you come home from school or work and you're *starving*, it can be difficult to look past the tempting bag of cookies or the delicious jar of chocolate spread rather than reach straight for your tin of mixed nuts. By keeping your food in a separate place, when the munchies strike, you won't be reaching for dried fruit while trying to overlook the bag of your favorite chips.

Being Surrounded by Negative Vibes: It can be challenging to create a healthy life you enjoy if those around you are constantly trying to bring you down. You work so hard day in and day out only to come home to negativity and harsh words. Or your co-workers constantly make you feel bad about the work and dedication you put toward your health. If you sit on the couch and complete watching a TV marathon of your favorite show, no one thinks twice. But order a salad over cheesecake and suddenly everyone is concerned about you and your life choices. It's ridiculous. Being healthy and active are *not* crimes and they're not "dangerous." Dedication is not synonymous with obsession. Dedication to your health and your goals does not equal mental illness. No one cared about my health (excluding my family) when I was overweight, but now that I am at a healthy weight, everyone and their mom has something to say. So how do you deal with that? How do you deal with all the extra and unwarranted "concern"?

I personally don't entertain people's comments and ideas about my health and my life. I'm a fitness instructor. I love to work out. I'm vegan, and I love fruits and vegetables! Taking strategic actions to ensure I have a healthy, active life is not anything to be ashamed of. And you shouldn't be ashamed or embarrassed either. Having scheduled workouts and prepping your meals will be so foreign to those who either 1) don't have a weight problem or 2) don't care about their health. And that is okay! Not everyone wants to be active and eat healthfully. To each their own! But I don't need to subject myself to claims from random negative people who have zero personal experience with what I grew up with. And neither do you.

If someone has never struggled with their weight or their health, they will not understand what it's like for an individual to completely transform their life in order to lose weight and improve their health. They will have zero understanding of the amount of dedication it takes to lose half your body weight. They will not understand *why* every workout is important, or how it's not just about the calories being burned, but also about the habits being formed. They won't understand how "skipping just this one day" can result in you deciding that the entire week will be a rest day. They won't understand the need to steer clear of tempting treats, and that just because something is your favorite treat does not mean you need it every chance you get. They won't understand these situations because weight is not something they have had to focus on.

Be intentional and create a healthy life around you. Find active buddies whom you can interact and build relationships with. Find people who share the same kinds of goals and health beliefs as you. Create a positive atmosphere around you. So when those negative people or individuals who just don't understand the struggles associated with weight loss try to bring you down or question your choices, the people who continue to support and encourage you through the tough times will surround you. Now I am not saying you should turn your nose up at all the sugary foods at a gathering or glare at people eating fast food. Everyone has a right to their preferences and that includes eating what they want. What I am saying is that you don't need to feel like an outcast for bringing a vegetable tray to a work gathering. You don't need to be ashamed that your favorite workout class is scheduled at the same time as happy hour, and that you would rather attend your class. Take pride in your goals and dream big! It's okay if people don't understand or believe in you. That's not your problem! It's theirs. Don't be influenced by negative people. Create a positive, uplifting life around you.

Significant-Other Opposites: I'm vegan. My husband is not. Some individuals have significant others who have drastically different eating habits, and this might cause major issues in their relationship. You might be married to a fast-food junkie or be dating a frozen-food-aisle champion. It can be challenging to have different eating styles, but it doesn't always have to be. You're an adult or young adult. Your significant other is too, and you can have different views on eating. People in healthy relationships encourage and support each other; they do not control each other. If your significant other wants to eat fried chicken for dinner, but you want baked chicken . . . is there a legitimate reason you can't both have what you want? In some cases, your significant other might want you to not only prepare your food, but also prepare their food. This is where I draw the line in my relationship. I am not a restaurant. I have no problem making side dishes that both Dre and I can enjoy, like steamed veggies, brown rice, and loaded vegetables with pasta. I love doing that! But what I can't do is prepare sides and two separate main dishes, such as baked tofu and his baked chicken. That becomes difficult in terms of eating dinner in a timely manner. So if this is you and your significant other, sit down together and create a plan. Do they like junk food? Great, they can eat it. But they have to be willing to help in the kitchen; after all, they're an adult too. You're their partner, not their mother.

This can cause tension in some relationships where cooking is seen solely as a one-person job. I get that. But again, you're not a restaurant. And it's not that you're *not* making dishes for your partner to enjoy, you're just being selective about your preparation of meals to ensure that mealtimes run smoothly and promptly. If your significant other wants fast food, they can eat it! But they shouldn't expect you to eat it too or to go pick it up for them. Encourage your family members to take responsibility for their eating habits.

I have friends who bend over backward for their spouses in terms of catering to their partners' food wants and needs. And that's okay! But if you're drained and it's putting a strain on your relationship, then a serious discussion needs to take place. You don't need to have matching food goals to make a relationship work. What you need is a common respect for each other's time and one another's food likes, dislikes, and choices.

In other relationships, though, it can be more complicated. For example, let's say you're worried about your significant other's health. Their eating habits are so damaging that their quality of life is being impacted. This is the person you want to spend the rest of your life with, but their choices have you worried about how long that life will be. And your health is also concerning. So you want to improve your health and lose weight to improve your quality of life, but your partner does not share the same passion or goals. So what can you do?

Have an honest heart-to-heart talk with them. Share your concerns and your fears. Share that you're worried about your significant other's health as well as your own, that you're troubled over how your food choices are impacting your children. Share your fears of raising kids with the current food and lifestyle choices you have. It can be a difficult conversation to have, but if it's important to you and your life, then it needs to take place. It's a conversation out of love, not judgment.

My husband and I have had many conversations about how we plan to raise our children when the time comes. Although I am vegan, Dre is not, and we have discussed what that will look like for our children. I will not raise our children vegan, because I feel it's a personal choice. But I will teach them the importance of healthy food choices. And when they get older they can decide for themselves what they would like to eat. We will have healthy food options in our house and encourage participation in daily activity, but I will not forbid my children to eat animal by-products.

Everyone will have a different view on raising children, but what is important is that you talk to your significant other about your goals, dreams, desires, and passions. If your significant other cannot support you in losing weight, then maybe some more steps need to be taken to help build that mutual respect for each other's goals.

Embracing Change: The situations mentioned above are harsh. You might be facing them right now, or you might face them later on in your journey. Mt. Weight Loss is not easy. It's not a few-weeks endeavor. You can't haphazardly jaunt up the path of successful weight loss. It's a life-altering experience that will reshape not only your body but also your entire life. And sometimes that reshaping process can be painful. Although the change is healthy and beneficial, change is still change. And as humans, we seem to have a natural aversion to any form of change. Even healthy change is a difficult concept to accept. The positive results of change can be staring you in the face and all you have to do is take a small step to reach them. And you will still find yourself hesitating, because it's a different course than what you're used to. You can see the top of Mt. Weight Loss—your goal weight and fitness aspirations are within your realm of control . . . and yet you hesitate to take the steps to reach them, because the process of change is involved. A different way of eating and thinking is required when traveling to your goals. This journey requires a different approach to life. And those differences—the change in mind-set, habits, and eating—prevent a lot of individuals from even attempting to start their journey. They are paralyzed by the fear of change, even though it could potentially save their life. Even though rock bottom is uncomfortable, miserable, and painful, the fear of change is more overwhelming to them than their current state of unhappiness.

It breaks my heart to see individuals so controlled by the fear of change and the unknown. I am saddened by the stories people share with me, about how they are exhausted with their current life circumstances. And how their rock bottom feels like it is gradually destroying their life. But they feel so helpless and hopeless because change is something they don't know if they can embrace. Their weight, in their eyes, is destroying any chance they have to live a happy life. But they would rather sit and weep every night about their weight than take a step in an unfamiliar direction. That is why I shove the importance of planning down your throat until you can't take it anymore.

A plan will give you the courage required to take the first step toward change. I don't care if you're tired of hearing the words "plan" and "structure." If you're on this journey for the long haul, you will need to get used to utilizing those skills every day. You cannot change your life without a structured plan.

That does not mean that every step you take must be premeditated and thoughtfully scrutinized. It merely means, for the love of all things holy, if you leave the house, grab an apple and a granola bar. You will get hungry, so be prepared. If you have a workout scheduled for 5:30 p.m., then go. You can't decide at the last minute that a movie sounds like a better idea. Planning, organizing, structuring, and scheduling: these are the skills that will help make change a concept that you can tackle. If you fear change you won't be successful on your journey. There will be lots of moments on your journey when you will have to change . . . and if you let your natural aversion to change prevent you from adapting and moving forward, your progress will be slow and you will unknowingly set up camp without ever reaching the top.

Embrace change. Your entire life is about to change, or currently is in the process of changing. It's okay to be uncomfortable, but learn to find comfort in your plan, your goals, and the excitement of taking control of your life. While this journey is hard, it's still marvelous and enjoyable! While I had my fair share of hard days, I've had more amazing experiences than negative ones. At the end of your journey, you will not remember the bad times; you will look back and everything will seem like a blur. You won't remember the time-consuming learning process of meal prep. All you will know is that you prep food like a professional. You won't remember the draining process of implementing daily exercise into your schedule. When you reflect back on your journey, it will seem like everything just fell into place naturally. But you will not wake up one day and—*bam!*—have magically reached your goal weight.

You will wake up day after day and be that much closer to your goal, until one day, when you wake up, you will realize that you no longer have to focus hard on reaching for healthy foods over junk. The habits you worked so hard on replacing will have seamlessly been replaced by healthy habits. Your healthy habits will have become second nature. Scheduled workouts will now be just a typical part of your day. A daily workout will no longer feel like a burden in your life.

The times you fought with all your heart and every ounce of self-control, those moments drove you to the top of the mountain. During the times you cried and groaned when pulling on your gym shoes, when life was beating you down and all you wanted to do was crawl back into bed and sleep forever, you didn't. You stuck to the course. You pressed on when everyone else would have sat down. You learned to say no to foods that would not feed your healthy side. And as a result everything you endured will seem worth it. You won't look back and think, "Wow, that was a wasted experience. I wish I hadn't worked so hard on taking control of my life and health."

You will look back and be overwhelmed with feelings of pride, gratefulness, empowerment, joy, and appreciation, as well as an overpowering sense of "I did it." Push through the change. Push through the tough times. You can make it through and you will only be that much stronger when you reach the other side.

Self-Isolation: When creating a healthy life and atmosphere it can be difficult to find a balance between friendship and your goals. It can be overwhelming to have people in your life who support both you and your goals . . . but still voice their negative opinions about your time commitments. Your first reaction might be to just cut ties with anyone who dares to question your dreams. So you end up cutting everyone who does not share the same healthy-living views as you out of your life, or you end all relationships with people who don't value the gym and exercise. That kind of cutthroat-friendship mentality is not healthy either. I've seen people completely isolate themselves in their own world of "health." Their entire life becomes centered on the gym, their reflection in the gym mirrors, food preparation, and the scale. That's not healthy and that is not what this journey is about.

A positive atmosphere is crucial to your journey but that does not mean you must isolate yourself and embrace all the challenges yourself. If someone close to you does not share your passion for weight loss, this does not mean that they can't still connect with you on your journey. You are chasing a goal. Lots of individuals chase goals. Whether these be educational goals, work-related goals, entrepreneur goals, etc., goal chasing is a commonality between lots of individuals. Just because a person does not have a weight-loss goal does not mean that they don't have *any* goals. While it's important to ensure you keep a close ring of positivity around you, this does not mean you need to host friendship interviews and associate yourself only with like-minded weight-loss-driven individuals. Branch out. Embrace differences. Find that healthy balance. This journey will take time, and when it comes to weight loss, you don't have to worry about "wasting" time. As long as the scale is moving in the right direction, you're golden.

9

Where Are the Rainbows and Unicorns?

I took one last deep breath and signaled to the class to slowly exhale. "Thank you, guys, for coming and have a great rest of your week if I don't see you tomorrow for Zumba!" I smiled to the class as I sent them out. The participants filed out of the room and I began to clean up and turn off the sound equipment. Typically, I feel unbelievable after teaching my favorite strength class. But today I felt so *blah*. I felt bloated, tired, and gigantic. My instructor shirt felt clingy and my arms looked puffy and toneless. I didn't even want to smile because my cheeks looked big and blotchy. "Just one of those days . . ." I groaned to myself as I grabbed my gym bag and began to make my way to the parking lot.

I said hi to a few people as I left the gym and decided that maybe a fresh fruit smoothie from the student café would make me feel better. I ordered the pineapple and coconut smoothie (one of my favorite combinations) and waited patiently to devour it. The girl working was a regular at my fitness classes and she quickly struck up a conversation with me. I put on my best fake smile while we talked and laughed as she made my smoothie. When it was ready, I thanked her and walked back to my car. I took one sip of my smoothie and threw it into the next garbage can I passed. It tasted great . . . but it wasn't what I wanted.

The tears began to well up in my eyes as I got inside my car. "Why do I feel like this?!" I began to cry to myself. "I work too hard to feel this bad about myself!"

The tears continued as I sat in my car. I pulled out my cell phone to call Dre. When he answered his phone the tears really began to pour. "What's wrong?" he gasped, with a lot of worry in his voice. "Are you okay?" he quickly asked. I assured him that I was okay, but that I was just having a really bad body day. I felt so stagnant with my weight loss and fitness, and I felt that I wasn't making any improvements with my body. I felt fat and uncomfortable with myself. Dre took a deep breath and then continued to try to soothe me, reassuring me that I was gorgeous and reminding me of how far I had come and how many people looked up to me because of what I had accomplished.

I knew he was right. But this made me feel even worse that I was so upset, and for no apparent reason apart from feeling "blah" about my body and myself. I hated it. I hated feeling that way! There I was with an amazing weight-loss story and a blog that continued to inspire hundreds of thousands of people daily. I was a fitness instructor who would encourage people every day, and I couldn't keep my own bad attitude at bay. I felt like such a hypocrite, which did not help to improve my already terrible mood.

I'm going to tell you right now that those "blah" days will happen more than once on your journey, and that they don't stop when you reach your goal weight. Reaching your goal weight does not prevent bad body-image days from occurring. Wearing your dream size does not prevent the "I feel fat and nothing fits" days. Crushing your fitness goals does not keep the bloat away. You *will* have bad days. There will be days when you cry over something stupid. There will be a day when you don't fit into the size that you think you should. There will be a time when you feel ugly and out of shape, regardless of how gorgeous and in shape you actually are! It happens! And it happens to the best of us. It does not mean that you're a failure at this whole "being fit thing," it just means you're human. No size, weight, or fitness ability can prevent bad days from happening or bad feelings from arising.

You will still have challenges when you reach your goals; you will just be smaller when you face them.

The best way to tackle those negative-feeling days is to have a wall of positivity that you can surround yourself with. This can be an actual motivational wall featuring other individuals and your own accomplishments, a place where you can proudly display your own "before" and "after" pictures. Or your wall of positivity can be figurative; it can be a person or a group of people whom you can call when you feel down and with whom you can be honest, people who don't expect you to pretend that you're okay when you're not. The hardest thing is pretending that you're not having a bad day when you're crushed inside. I can do that for only so long before it starts to actually make me feel worse! While faking a smile can improve some bad days, other times you need to be honest and find someone whom you can talk things out with.

Brea and I had plenty of late-night talks when I had bad days. We would sit on my bed and watch baking shows while we vented about our current mind-sets, our day, and our blah body image. Some days I felt terrible about school and I needed to complain about it. My master's program was incredibly difficult, and some of my classmates made the schoolwork seem so easy. But for me, schoolwork has always been challenging. I had to give 110 percent just to get an average grade. It was so frustrating. Add bad school days to blah body days, and I was a blubbering mess.

Thank God that I had Brea and Dre to handle all my late-night phone calls and chats. And my mom was always there on the horrendous days too. Because on days when you really feel that your life is in shambles, like the day I failed an important exam, those are days that require a call to Mom. Life happens. Bad days are going to happen! But you don't have to let the bad days ruin you, and you don't have to dive into a pint of your favorite ice cream in order to feel better. So you have a bad day. Your entire life will not be shaped by this one day.

Unfortunately, I had unrealistic expectations about reaching my goal weight. I thought everyone would think I was the prettiest person and flock to me. I thought I could wear anything I wanted and rock it. I thought I would look like a model and be treated like a fantasy girl. Sounds pretty ridiculous and vain, right? But I *know* I am not the only person who has thought this way. This whole book is about my honest experience with the good and the bad, so these are my candid thoughts. I thought life would be perfect once I lost a hundred pounds, and I was wrong. I thought I would find happiness at the end of my journey, and I was mistaken.

I reached my goal and I had bad days. I had days when I felt ugly. I had days when I felt fat. I did not have random people begging for my attention. I had to ask for larger sizes in dressing rooms. I tried on trendy clothes and looked ridiculous. I had to return clothes people bought me as gifts because they purchased a size too small. I had days when my cellulite really bothered me. I couldn't walk around the house in a tiny nightie and feel confident around my husband every night. I didn't walk around the kitchen in my underwear and make pancakes for him. I couldn't put on a bikini and wash my car any day of the week. I didn't get asked if I was a model. I wasn't pulled out of lines at nightclubs and given VIP treatment. I didn't feel confident in any shirt I put on.

I had all these ideas about what it would feel like to reach my goal weight . . . and when I finally got there . . . and all those things didn't happen . . . it was a rude awakening! It made me feel like I hadn't tried hard enough, that I could have been doing more! I was in the best shape of my life and *still* felt like it wasn't enough. Having unrealistic expectations can do that to you. They set you up to feel bad even after accomplishing something incredible. I worked hard to lose all that weight, but I was left feeling frustrated that my life was not perfect, that my body was not perfect.

Don't get me wrong, I am not trying to be a downer, and I certainty don't want to detour anyone from reaching their goals! Climbing Mt. Weight Loss is one of the biggest accomplishments of my life. What I am trying to share is that your life won't be perfect when you reach the top. And if you expect nothing but perfection when you reach your goals, then you will be disappointed. That disappointment can lead to a slow and steady descent back down the mountain, a.k.a. weight gain.

And I'm not talking a five- to ten-pound fluctuation, I am talking about a steady forty-five-plus-pound weight gain, to the point where you are practically back at your rock bottom. It happens more often than you think. And you might be reading this and realizing that this is why you are climbing up Mt. Weight Loss—again. Unrealistic expectations set you up for realistic letdowns.

I thought that when I reached my goal weight I would feel confident all the time. That every day, 24/7, I would ooze with confidence and be able to be that girl who could throw on a pair of tight jeans and a simple tank and leave the house looking flawless . . .Yeah, I'm still not that girl. It takes me a few minutes to get the whole "flawless" look. For a while I was frustrated that I didn't feel "perfect," until I realized that reaching a goal weight does not equal perfection. I will always have parts of my body that I want to improve, and I can either choose to be happy or choose to chase the never-ending quest for perfection. Now that I understand that my life is a work in progress versus a completed project, I am much happier. I still have blah days, but I don't have "my life is terrible days" anymore. That might sound a bit dramatic, but you will relate when it happens to you, when you feel like you wasted your whole summer by exercising and eating healthfully but still feel out of shape and unattractive. It happens. There is no finish line filled with cheering, adoring fans who want to shower you with never-ending compliments and praise. There is no social club you join to meet other equally attractive singles. There is no perfect clothing line that makes everything you ever wanted to wear in the perfect, most flattering fit. These are unrealistic expectations of what reaching the top of Mt. Weight Loss entails. The love of your life is not waiting for you at the top of Mt. Weight Loss. And the sooner you understand that, the less disappointed you will be when you complete the climb.

There are no rainbows and unicorns at the top. Your problems don't vanish when you reach your goal size. When you get to the top you won't instantly find happiness and self-love. In fact, the attitude you develop while climbing Mt. Weight Loss is the attitude you will have when you reach the top. If you hate the climb, you will hate the top. If you hate your body and constantly focus on your imperfections, when you reach the end of the climb, you will continue to focus on the negative and have a bad attitude.

A positive attitude and healthy habits are necessities for a lasting healthy life. I'm not saying you will be happy all the time, as my own experiences with bad days demonstrate. What I am saying is that by choosing a positive attitude you can help shape your journey and life to be a positive experience. So when those bad days happen—and they will—you can deal with them and then move on. I've had my fair share of letdowns. But I don't dwell on them, I grow from them. And I move on. That's all you can do in life! Either you grow or you descend back down. You never stay the same.

So the next time a bad day strikes, handle it the best you can and then move on. Just because you had a bad day . . . you don't have a bad life. And this is not the whole "suck it up because someone elsewhere has it worse than you" philosophy. That statement does not help anybody. You have every right to be upset, frustrated, and angry. It's all relative! But understand this: being upset, frustrated, and angry will not solve your problems. While your feelings are valid, they are not the solution. Grow from the situation, don't dwell on it. Experience whatever emotions you have and then focus on developing a solution. It's not the end of the world, just a bump in the road.

So how do you overcome the lack of rainbows and unicorns? Well, life can still be great without being perfect. You have your health, for one thing. And you *did* reach your goals, or are on your way to reaching your goals. Since when is that a bad thing? I'm not saying you will never have good days. What I am saying is that you will have bad days mixed in with the good days. You won't wake up every day in a fantastic mood. Every day won't be a skintight-clothes day. You're going to have baggy-clothes days, bad-body-image days, bloated days, fluffy days, and all-of-the-above days. But again, that doesn't mean you won't have amazing days too! Life is full of dynamics. If every day were amazing, amazing would become the norm and things would stop being amazing. Amazing would become the new average. You need the variations in your life to truly appreciate how wonderful life really is. You don't see rainbows on days when the sky is blue and filled with sunshine. You see rainbows after a storm has passed and the sun begins to peek through the dark clouds. *Wait out the storms, because the rainbows are about to make their grand entrance.*

Let's address some individual unrealistic expectations. The first one is, *the scale will never change when you reach your goal weight*. False. The scale will change every day. You can weigh yourself three times a day and see a different number each time. That is why I have always opted for a healthy weight range versus a specific number. While I fully support having a set goal-weight number or ultimate goal weight, establishing a healthy weight range allows my goal to be more realistic and attainable in the long run. The scale can be affected by numerous non-weight-related factors: water retention, sodium intake, muscle swelling, hormones, etc. If you allow the scale to determine the type of day you're going to have, you're going to have quite a few bad days. Aim for a goal range and weigh yourself once a week or every other week. The scale should be used only to determine if you're on track, not to determine your happiness. And eventually, you won't even need the scale. When you're living an active and healthy life, your weight will take care of itself.

Another common unrealistic expectation is *clothing size*. When I go shopping at the mall, I can vary between a size one and a size nine; it depends on the clothing store. And if I were to measure my worth or success by the size of clothing I buy, my mood would be all over the place. Some stores would make me feel fantastic and other stores would leave me feeling miserable. So what is more important to focus on? How you look in the clothes. How the clothes make you feel. So what if the dress that fits you is a large? You look fantastic in it! It hugs your body in all the right places and makes you feel ready for a night out. No one knows the size of your clothes but you, and even then, it still doesn't matter. If you want to have a "dream size," I suggest picking one brand or store and using it as your guide. If you set your goal to be the same size clothing in all brands, you are looking for a unicorn. It's not going to happen. You will not be a size five in every brand. That is unrealistic.

What is a more realistic clothing-related goal? To look good in jeans, that's a good goal. I did not wear jeans until I weighed in the 160s.

Before, jeans did not make me feel good. Any pair of jeans I wore prior to losing weight quickly developed holes in the inner-thigh seam because my legs rubbed together. Talk about an awesome boost for your self-confidence—a daily reminder that you're so overweight you cause clothes-ruining friction just from walking. Eventually, I joined the leggings-as-pants movement and stopped wearing jeans altogether. I vividly remember buying my first pair of single-digit-size jeans. It was such a rush! Have realistic expectations and your journey will be much more enjoyable. Have a goal to feel comfortable in clothes, regardless of size. Right this moment I am wearing size-two jeans, but if I tried that in some other stores, I wouldn't even be able to get the pants past my calves! My goal was to rock a pair of jeans, not worry about the size on the label.

Another common unrealistic expectation is that *all clothing styles will look good on you*. False. When you lose weight, your body shape changes. Before I lost weight, I had a pretty decent hourglass shape. Although I carried weight in my stomach, because I was tall, my weight was evenly distributed throughout my body. I also had large breasts. Yeah, I don't have those anymore. I have since joined the itty-bitty-titty committee. Dresses that were tight at the waist and flared at the hips used to look good on me. Now I need more structure along my hips or else I look like I have a boyish frame. My hips are now wider than my upper torso (since my boobs volunteered for the weight-loss process) and I have a hard time balancing the upper and lower halves of my body, disproportions that I had never dealt with before. I can't just go grab anything off the rack and expect that I am going to rock it. I have to try things on just like everyone else.

You will still have to try clothes on and shop for your shape. It might be a new shape, or be a similar shape to what you currently have, just smaller. But you will still need to shop with a purpose. Shopping is more enjoyable for me now and I have more options, but I can't wear every style on the market. Drop-waist maxi dresses and A-line skirts are not flattering on my new body. But I do look great in body-con dresses and pencil skirts. Rainbows will not continually be arching at the shopping mall when you reach your goal weight. You will still find yourself flustered in the dressing room and throwing clothes on the floor in the morning. You're changing your weight, not the structure of the known clothing universe.

Another misconception is that *when you reach your goal weight, attractive people will flock to you and instantly adorn you with their love.* Okay, so maybe that sounds a bit extreme, but I am sure you have found yourself daydreaming once or twice about how nice it would be if you were thin so your crush would notice you. Or about how it would feel to be the "hot" friend who gets all the attention. Truth is, there are not crowds of singles waiting to love you once you reach your goal weight. There is no hot club you instantly earn a membership to when you can squeeze into your goal dress size. Shrinking your body does not move you up on the universal scale of attractiveness.

People are attracted to all different body types. I am currently too thin for some people and not thin enough for others. I have people who think I have too much muscle on me and others who tell me that I look "skinny-fat." I'm either too bony or too muscular. But honestly, I already found the love of my life, so I personally don't care how attractive other people find me.

But you might not be with the love of your life. You might be waiting until you reach your goal weight so everyone will find you attractive, if you even want to fall in love . . . It just doesn't work that way. Your body type will not be attractive to 100 percent of the world's population. Some people will love your new body, and other people might say that you looked better with "meat on your bones." You will always be too thin, too fat, too scrawny, too muscular, too *whatever* for all different kinds of people!

So what is important is that you love you. You decide what you want to look like. Don't leave that up to other people, and don't expect everyone to appreciate the hard work you put into your goals, because not everyone will. This is my least favorite topic to write about because I make it seem depressing to reach your goals. It's not, I promise. But there are certain unrealistic expectations people can have when they set out to reach their goals. If they don't accept that it just doesn't work that way, they will be incredibly disappointed when they reach the top of Mt. Weight Loss—that is, if they even make it to the top.

Some people are so crushed by the weight of the letdown of their expectations that they let it prevent them from ever reaching the top. I met my husband while I was on my weight-loss journey. I was 230 pounds when Dre and I met. I was not even close to my goal. But what improved over the course of my first twenty-pound loss were my confidence and appreciation for my goals and myself. That is what Dre found most attractive about me, my perseverance to reach my goals. And he joined me on my journey and ended up reaching his own weight-loss goals. When Dre and I got married I was literally half the person he fell in love with. But he fell in love with me, not my body type. Your change in body type won't help you find the love of your life, your Prince Charming, or your Beauty Queen. Having confidence and loving yourself will help you continue to push yourself to reach your goals. And who knows whom you will meet along the way! Not everyone will love the new you, the old you, or the current you. So what is important is that *you* love you!

Here's another unrealistic expectation: *when you reach your goal weight you can eat whatever you want and be fine.* False. You will always need to be conscious of your food choices. You are adopting a healthy lifestyle, not a diet. And if you begin to think that you no longer need to pay attention to your food choices, you will slowly descend back down Mt. Weight Loss. There is a lot of research to support that individuals who lose substantial amounts of weight can't keep it off. Why is that? It's because of the diet mentality, the mentality that "I will eat a certain way until I am thin, and then I can go back to eating 'normally.'" It just doesn't work that way! And if you think that reaching your goal weight guarantees you a spot in the "thin life," then you are in for a really rude wake-up call.

Healthy is for life. And if you're not ready to accept that, then the climb up Mt. Weight Loss is just not for you. You won't be able to successfully complete your journey. I don't need to be a certified life coach or a dietitian to know that. You *have* to live a healthy life past reaching your goal if you want to maintain your weight. You *will* gain weight if you don't accept that.

Individuals who diet only to reach their goals are the ones who gain it back. People who change their lives for the better and become healthier individuals are the ones who maintain their weight loss. It's the hard truth. If you think you will be "done" living the healthy life when you reach your goal weight and you can't wait to binge-eat pizza every night with your friends again, then you won't stay at your goal weight for longer than a week. It's unrealistic to expect your body to stay at a healthy weight while you lead an unhealthy life. Your eating habits enabled you to reach your lowest point in the first place. Remember your rock-bottom moment? How can you expect temporary changes to lead to permanent results? That's unrealistic.

Does that mean you can never have treats and splurges? Absolutely not. Enjoy your date nights and ice cream sundae parties with your friends. But be prepared to order a side salad over fries more often, and don't feel the need to reach for the cookie tray every day at work. Is that a bad thing, though? I don't think so. Why should it be bad to want to live healthier? My body feels better when I eat a bowl of fresh cut strawberries over a handful of candy anyway. And your body will too. Being healthy is not a punishment. Healthy eating should not be viewed as an aversion therapy technique for fat. Enjoy your treats and your Sunday morning cinnamon roll tradition, but also enjoy healthy foods, like fresh fruits, vegetables, whole grains, and less-processed foods. I think this is about the tenth time I have made this point, but it is just so important: how your body loses the weight is how your body learns to maintain it. So what are you teaching your body? What are you learning during this process? Is it something you can maintain?

Another common goal-reaching misconception is that *exercise will be easy and I will always want to do it.* False. Super false! I'm a fitness instructor and there are days when the only reason I complete a workout is that it's my job and I have to be there. Exercise will not always be something you strive to do. And if you're waiting for that moment when the addiction to exercise hits you . . . you're going to be waiting a while. While there are times I crave a good endorphin rush, it's not 24/7. There are days I am so tired that all I want to do is sleep. Days when all I want to do is eat. Days when all I want to do is binge-watch my favorite TV show and cuddle up with my dog, Tofu.

Exercise can become a habit and a regular part of your routine, but it will always be challenging regardless of how ingrained it becomes. Exercise does not become easier, you simply become stronger. That is why it's so important to find a type of exercise that you enjoy. Otherwise, exercise will become daunting, and not only will you not want to exercise, you will also hate every minute of it. Exercise has become one of my stress outlets (exercise and buying coffee are my two stress relievers), but I also have days when I dread going to the gym. It just happens! Not every day will be a fantastic day. When you reach your goal weight, you will not feel prepped and ready to run a marathon every morning.

There have been times when I have been in the middle of a workout and tears will begin to form in my eyes, not because I am in pain, but because I am so done with the gym or the workout video. But I have to push through. I have to remain physically and mentally strong. Because although I am so frustrated with exercise that I am on the verge of tears, my goals depend on my ability to persevere even on those emotional days. It's in those times that I think back to my days with my personal trainer, and I can hear her voice in my head challenging me to keep going: "Keep pushing. You can do this."

If every time I listened to that inner voice that told me, "Just this once take a rest day," I would not have reached my goals. I did take rest days, don't get me wrong. But my body does not need six rest days a week. And that is what would have happened if I had listened to that voice. It's unrealistic to believe that wanting to exercise will always come naturally to you; exercise will always take work. But the amount of work it takes is dependent on how much you enjoy your exercise routine. Find a fitness style you love and it will feel less like "work." It is the whole idea of "I get to" versus "I have to." Again, exercising won't always be the best time of your life and you will want to skip it on numerous occasions, but push through. Understanding that it's normal to want to skip on fitness will help you through the post-weight-loss process.

So what is the post-weight-loss process? Well, once you understand that rainbows and unicorns are not waiting for you when you reach your goals, you might experience a "what's next?" emotion. This is that feeling of not being sure what you're doing with your life anymore. You have worked so hard to reach a goal, and now that you have reached it . . . you are left feeling empty—fulfilled and excited, but empty, nonetheless. I've been there.You might be there right now. And for others, that feeling will come a little later on. The first time I experienced it, it left me feeling down and mission-less. I knew I didn't want to keep losing weight. But I wanted to keep working toward something, and if not weight loss, then what?

I was left searching for a new goal that I could chase. My new goal was to share my story with as many people as possible. I was no longer the focus of my journey. I wanted to share my story and passion for health and fitness.

That is when I fully dived into group fitness and blogging. I also developed more challenging fitness goals. I tried different forms of exercise and pushed myself beyond my comfort zone with new workout programs. It's important to set goals for yourself and to continually invest in your health and life. Sometimes when people reach the end of their journey, they stop. They stop going to the gym and they stop buying healthy foods. The post-weight-loss adrenaline rush wears off and they are left feeling lost, empty, and goal-less. That is why it's so important to continually build up your support circle of positivity around you, so when you reach your goals, you have other people who can help you establish new goals and dreams to pursue.

Take this time to reflect on your own personal expectations for when you reach your goal weight. Are they realistic? Or are you unknowingly chasing a unicorn and hoping for rainbows 24/7? While you will be stronger, healthier, and happier once you reach your goals, it's important to fully understand that losing weight will not solve all your problems. Skills are learned and earned along the journey, based on how hard you focused on developing them. Happiness is waiting for you at the top of the mountain. But you have to choose it while making the climb.

Check off the expectations that you have for when you reach your goal:

- ☐ Finding perpetual happiness
- ☐ Feeling self-love
- ☐ Finding Prince Charming
- ☐ Feeling the yearning to exercise 24/7
- ☐ No longer needing to "diet"
- ☐ Having the perfect body for clothes
- ☐ Size of clothes no longer mattering
- ☐ Receiving constant attention from attractive people
- ☐ Being perceived to have the perfect body by others
- ☐ Becoming someone's "dream girl" or "dream guy"
- ☐ Other: ________________________________

Now based on the expectations you checked, are you searching for a unicorn? Do you dream of the days when your life will constantly be filled with rainbows? Are you setting yourself up for a positive post-weight-loss experience? Or are you creating a path toward frustration, letdown, and difficult weight management once you reach your goal? Are your expectations realistic? Why or why not?

____

____

____

If your expectations are in the fields with the unicorns, what are some more realistic expectations you can focus on?

____

____

____

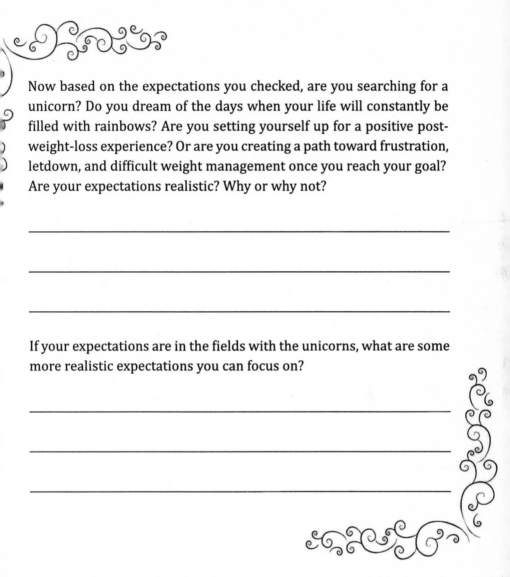

10

You're Busy, I Get It

School is kicking your butt. All you can think about are the copious amounts of homework and due dates that haunt you when you try to sleep. Your boss is throwing more on your plate, and at this point you don't even have time to schedule bathroom breaks let alone schedule a workout. You can't blow your nose without fear of losing a precious moment to study for your upcoming exam. The very thought of taking a break causes clinical levels of anxiety. So how do you deal with that? How can you possibly exercise when you don't even have enough time to sleep? You. Don't. Have. Time.

I've been there. I've been the graduate student in a position where the only good excuse to miss class was if I were on my deathbed. And I've had to sit through a few classes where I was so sick, I thought I *was* on my deathbed! I've been so overwhelmed with school I just wanted to cry and pray everything away. So how can you stay on track when all you want to do is weep and give up? Take a step back and breathe. You can't accomplish anything if you're running around like a chicken with its head cut off. You can't reach your goals if you're sitting in the back in fetal position. Nothing can be accomplished if your lens for the world is predicting failure, doom, and immediate demise.

Focus on what you can control. You can't control your hectic school demands and you can't control the tasks your boss decides to put on your plate. You have to go to class and you have to fulfill your student requirements. You have to go to work and you have to accomplish your daily work demands. And you have to eat. Now, which "have to" most contributes to your weight? What you put in your body. Your food choices impact your weight the most. And guess what you have the most control over? Your food choices. Groundbreaking, right?

What do you find yourself reaching for when those stressful moments arise? Let's look at a couple scenarios. We will call the crazy-stressed person in scenario one "Alex." When Alex is cramming for a test, she reaches for apple slices and peanut butter. When asked to stay late at work, she orders a vegetable sub from a local deli. When the late-night munchies hit, she has mixed nuts with coconut shreds. When she is running late for class in the morning, she grabs a quick bowl of oatmeal topped with fresh berries and peanut butter granola chunks.

Let's call crazy-stressed person in scenario two "Josh." When Josh is rushing to complete a ten-page essay he procrastinated on, he orders pizza and soda for him and his roommates. When asked to volunteer at a work event, he hangs out by the dessert bar all night. When rushing to school in the morning, Josh stops at a nearby fast-food joint for some quick-and-easy breakfast wraps. When the late-night cravings hit, he shops the candy aisle and stocks up on all his favorites.

Now do you think Alex and Josh, who are both stressed and insanely busy, would experience the same weight issues? Absolutely not. When you're super stressed and feel like your life is falling apart, focus on your food. You have control over what you put in your body. Food is powerful. It's how our bodies live. It's our fuel. Make the right choices starting at the grocery store and you will have the tools to help control your crazy life. Will this get you straight A's and a promotion at work? Probably not. But you will not feel your pants getting tighter, and you might even find yourself having to squeeze in time to buy a smaller size. I think I could handle that kind of stress.

Food is such an underutilized tool for weight control and weight loss. Exercise is incredibly important and beneficial for overall health.

But sometimes, exercise is just not something people can physically or mentally commit to. And that is okay. But you will always have to eat regardless of time. Food is non-negotiable. It's an everyday, multiple-times-a-day event! If you find yourself unable to commit to exercise right now, that is okay. Focus on what you can commit to—food. If your health, for whatever reason, such as an injury or medical condition, prevents you from incorporating exercise into your daily life, start your healthy-life transformation with food. What you put in your body will have a direct relationship with your weight, whether good or bad. Eat healthy foods, and healthy things will happen to your body. Eat unhealthy things, and continue to have negative health issues arise. Every time you walk into the doctor's office, your weight will be mentioned. Wouldn't it be nice to walk into the doctor's office and not dread the scale? Or not have to face the feared conversation about how your BMI is not within a healthy range?

Far too often people procrastinate on shifting to a healthy lifestyle because of time constraints. They want to be healthy and they have goals to change their life, but . . . they figure they'll change their life eventually, just not right at this moment, with excuses such as "This is just not a good time for me" or "Maybe next week, when I can plan better" or the super popular "I will start on Monday." However, even individuals with crazy schedules still eat. You have to eat. But it's a matter of *what* you eat, not *if* you eat. Here's a tough-love moment for you: your health is not fascinated with how important your reasons for not losing weight are. No excuse is ever good enough to justify lack of responsibility for your health.

It takes just as much time to reach for an apple as it does for a bag of chips. You can cook a bowl of oatmeal in the same amount of time it would take to heat up a frozen breakfast burrito. What stops people from starting their journey is not the time constraint, but the fear of the unknown. Not knowing what foods to buy or what foods are considered healthy is scary. Grocery stores are large. And if you don't know what to purchase, you will find yourself continually purchasing the same unhealthy foods or just sticking to fast food, especially if you're stressed. Who wants to revamp their life when they feel like their life is already unmanageable? If you're functioning on limited sleep, the last thing you want to do is focus any brain energy on what foods you should eat. So you stick with what you know, even if your waistline is pleading for you to reconsider your choices. Denial can last for only so long. Eventually, you will have to face your food choices. Don't wait until it's too late.

Another fear and commonly used weight-loss-journey-halting excuse is money. Can you afford to eat healthfully? What will it do to your budget? I can assure you that, after having been in college for eight years, it is possible to eat healthfully on a tight budget. Produce and whole-grain products go on sale too. Search for the deals. And you don't need to purchase the $15 loaf of dragon's breath whole-grain sprouted bread that was blessed by the pope himself. The generic brand of whole-wheat bread is good for you too. It's all about shopping smart. You don't have to get sucked into the fad brands, and you don't need to purchase everything organic (unless you want to). I lost all my weight with very few organic purchases. I bought healthy, whole foods without my progress being halted by what was on food labels. Shop smart and don't fall victim to marketing scams. Healthy food does not have to equal an expensive budget. The fear of going broke should not prevent you from changing your life. It's a common fear, but it's avoidable.

It comes down to two options: either continuing to be a ball of stress and gaining weight, or continuing to be a ball of stress who loses weight. You *can* control your food choices without completely altering your entire schedule. And you don't need to be a walking encyclopedia of nutrition in order to navigate the grocery store. Stick to the basics: fresh fruits and vegetables, whole grains, lean proteins, and healthy fats. Avoid conventional unhealthy foods like cookies, cake, chips, anything fried, etc. Stop purchasing the foods that you know are not good for you. If you keep good foods in your house, you will be less tempted to purchase fast food on your way to work or school. If you shop smart, you will have all the healthy foods you need to conquer your day. Again, healthy food won't fix all your problems, but it will give you a sense of control over your weight. Toast with peanut butter topped with banana slices takes six minutes max to make. You're telling me that a fast-food drive-through can make your meal in a shorter amount of time than that? Time is not the problem. It's fear that is holding you back. You can learn to eat healthy food. It's an adjustment. But don't blame work, school, or time as a reason that you can't start your journey right now. You can.

This is another tough-love topic for me. It's a tough-love section because I've been there. I lost my weight while in college. I lived on a tight budget, was stressed out, and was short on time. But I still managed to completely change my life and reach my goals. I became that person who brought her lunch to school. I packed my protein bars and peanut butter whole-wheat sandwiches. I carried my apple slices with me and snacked during breaks. If I went to the cafeteria with friends, I searched for the whole-wheat options and actually used the school salad bar. Initially, people questioned why I was eating healthfully and commented on how my food seemed "boring." But eventually, those same people wanted to know exactly what I was doing, because they noticed my progress. They saw the results I was getting and wanted to do what I did. They wanted to eat the same things I ate, they wanted to learn more about the vegan diet, and they wanted to attend the same exercise classes I went to.

You will find that in your life too. Those who question you will want to follow you if you give the process enough time. Change takes time. So if you're so incredibly stressed that your life can't handle an overhaul of both food and activity right now, start with food. Focus on that. Food can drastically change your life for the better. I promise.

Stop frequenting the drive-through and prepare your meals before you leave the house. Your health and wallet will thank you in the long run. I would turn on my favorite TV show the night before and prepare my meals and snacks for the next day. It's all about priorities. Food preparation did take me a few weeks to get the hang of; sometimes I did not prepare enough food or I made too much and it spoiled quickly. But those are things you learn along the way—you will learn the things that work and the things that don't! The longer you go without junk food, though, the easier it will be to overcome the urge to eat it. If you're constantly filling up on healthy foods, you won't have the space to eat unhealthy foods.

When it comes to preparing foods, a major component is planning to ensure you have enough time to prep. This also comes down to priorities. I know stress is why you choose to focus solely on food. But food preparation is important, so it's one of those areas where I just have to say, "Make it work." It does not take long to adjust your routine to include food preparation. If you want to add brown rice into your diet, make large batches on Sunday night and then pre-portion the rice into plastic containers. That way it's just a matter of grabbing a container when you're ready to leave for work or school.

I typically make large batches of foods on Sunday night. That gives me a chance to see what my week will look like, and I can plan accordingly. I've been food-prepping for years now, so it's a skill I've developed well. So be patient with yourself. It will take time to become a seasoned food-prepper, but you will get there. Just like with anything else, the more you practice, the stronger the skill becomes. Don't be discouraged if it takes you a while to get the hang of it. Time is one of the hardest components of food preparation to understand. And when you're already short on time, dedicating yourself to your goals will help you *make* time to prep your food. Remember, no one can lose the weight for you. Only you can make the necessary changes to reach them.

You're beyond stressed. And this whole chapter might be making you stress out even more! But your health is important. You can't control the craziness in your life, but you can control your food choices. You have to grocery shop at some point during the week, so go with a plan—make a list and stick to it! Think simple; you're not out to make five-star gourmet meals. If you watch their sodium content, you can find some great canned soups that are perfect for lunch. Find some soup and pair it with a vegetable-loaded salad or a lean-protein-and-vegetable-loaded wrap. Healthy does not have to mean plain rice cakes and mounds of steamed vegetables (although I do love my vegetables). Find a cookbook that speaks to you and look through it for ideas. When I was in school I ate peanut butter whole-wheat sandwiches with fresh raspberries in place of jam. I paired the sandwich with chopped apples and pears. Filling, healthy, easy, and cheap—every college student's dream!

Healthy does not have to be debilitating or cumbersome. You can reach your goals and still maintain a functioning work and school life. There will be a readjustment period, but that does not last forever. Like I said, you have to eat. You have to grocery shop. So make healthy choices with your food and you will be that much closer to reaching your goals.

11

Birth of the *A Funeral for My Fat* Blog

It was another night and I was having difficulty falling asleep. I was only a few months away from graduating with my bachelor's degree and my senioritis was on full blast. I aimlessly searched through social media on my phone, catching up on the drama of all my old friends from high school. I was at a good place in my weight loss, and old friends I hadn't seen in a while were continually commenting on the pictures I would post and saying how great I looked. Eventually, while on a routine social media dive, I stumbled upon some weight-loss blogs.

I began reading post after post of weight-loss tips and helpful advice. There were inspiring "before" and "after" pictures that motivated me to continue on my own journey. But soon after stumbling on the weight-loss community blogs, I found a deeper and darker side. I began to read stories of girls eating less than 250 calories a day in order to have a thigh gap. I saw pictures of girls with their bones jutting out from their skin, and below the pictures the girls would say, "Ugh, I feel so fat today." I found tips on how to not feel hungry during the day, and how to beat hunger pangs and live off only water. What shocked me the most was not the content, but the number of people who appeared to think this was good advice. The comments that followed typically said things like "Wow, great advice, thanks for sharing!" and "This is something I've got to try—I'm so fat!"

I felt sick. How could people read this and think it was the way to weight loss?! I read post after post in disbelief. Some posts promoting starvation-type techniques had thousands of comments on them—and they weren't comments sharing in my disbelief. They were comments of people actually wanting to implement the "advice." The more I read, the more angry, sad, and repulsed I felt. It was like a train wreck; I couldn't stop looking at it, reading the comments and staring at picture after picture of individuals with severe (and self-proclaimed) eating disorders who were sharing their weight-loss "advice." For a whole week, every night, I would go look at the pictures and see what new posts and "advice" were posted. Even though I was sickened by it, I was drawn to it. It was about weight loss. And no matter how much I tried to stay away from it, my curiosity got the best of me. *What are they posting today? What pictures did they post as "inspiration" today?* I found myself thinking.

Here I was, a twenty-one-year-old woman who had found herself sucked into blogs promoting anorexia out of pure curiosity. It wasn't because I wanted to be like that, but because this was an online world centrally focused on weight loss. And that was what I was on a mission to do, lose weight. But not this way. I was already down ninety-one pounds. Weight loss was nothing new to me. But I didn't have an outlet for my weight loss, an online world that was centrally concentrated on losing weight . . . Until now. But it left me sick, sad, and disheartened, not motivated, inspired, or happy. But it was about weight loss. So I kept going back.

My curiosity did not last long. Eventually, my heart became too burdened by the number of people influenced by the sites. I knew weight loss could be achieved by healthy means, but after viewing these popular blogs, it was glaringly evident that not everyone knew that. People actually believed that by attempting to develop an eating disorder and by miming habits of those with disorders, they could reach their weight-loss goals and achieve their dream body. Individuals talked about eating disorders and severe dieting as if this were just common practice, the norm for sustainable weight loss. I couldn't take it anymore. I did not create a blog to change the diet culture or silence the anorexia "diet" supporters. I created a blog to have a place to share my story—a healthy weight-loss story.

The name "A Funeral for My Fat" occurred to me as I was trying to come up with a catchy title for my blog, something that made me laugh but also demonstrated the permanence of my approach and philosophy to weight loss. And what is more permanent than death? When something dies, it doesn't come back. I had zero intentions of ever needing to lose over one hundred pounds again! I started my blog and posted my very first "before" and "after" pictures. Within a few minutes of my picture posting, I began to receive messages in my inbox asking me how I lost the weight. I began to answer questions daily. I posted regularly and my audience began to grow. People wanted to know how I lost the weight. What I ate. What exercise I did. How I stayed motivated. All of these topics that I had had to find out for myself, I was now able to share with people who were experiencing the same types of things I experienced.

Every person will create a different path up Mt. Weight Loss, one that works for them. Healthy is healthy. Motivational tips are motivational tips. People wanted to hear firsthand how I dealt with the highs and lows of weight loss. How I handled my urges to overeat. How I ate at restaurants and managed to stay on track. My blog became a central movement during the online shift from pro-eating-disorder blogs to pro-healthy-living blogs. I wanted to share that you can eat *enough* and still lose weight. You can enjoy exercise. You don't need to be a runner to look like a runner. You don't need to spend three hours a day at the gym in order to reach your goals. I shared my story, my pictures, and my advice, and the response was incredible.

My blog seemingly grew from having a few hundred follows to hundreds of thousands in a few months. My inbox became so flooded with questions that I could no longer answer them. I began developing quick-link guides to address frequently asked questions and situations people find themselves facing. My blog always focused on two things: health and happiness, choosing to be healthy and choosing to be happy. It became a central location where individuals could find daily motivation and healthy eating tips, and hear from a person who was on the same journey as them.

When I first started my journey up Mt. Weight Loss, I didn't have one person I could talk to who had reached the top. I had friends who enjoyed exercise, and I always had my mom by my side, but this was not the same as being able to see someone's progress and hear their advice regarding the exact same things I was experiencing. I wanted advice on motivation. I wanted to learn how to eat healthfully on a college student budget. I wanted to know what the best types of foods to eat were. I was curious about what losing massive amounts of weight would feel like. The emotions you experience on the way are numerous. Does it ever get easier? What does it feel like to look in the mirror and be "small"? So many questions, and I didn't have anyone who could answer them.

I had magazine stories that I had saved and hung up on my bedroom wall, stories about people who ran themselves to their goal weight or individuals who walked away fifty pounds. These were all inspiring, and well-written articles. But I couldn't talk to the people the articles were about. I couldn't ask them to describe in detail their rock-bottom moments. I couldn't pick their brain on what the best foods to eat were. I couldn't ask what losing over a hundred pounds felt like, and whether their life was perfect now. I didn't have a single person—I had cutout magazine stories taped to a bulletin board in my room! Pictures of real people can be motivating too, don't get me wrong! But I wanted to feel a relationship. I wanted to see a "real" person who had lost the weight and hear from them about their daily struggles. My blog became that "real" person to others who were in the same place I had been in three years earlier, trying to lose massive amounts of weight and feeling alone on the journey because no one around me was on a journey to lose a hundred-plus pounds.

I wanted to offer a place where others could vent their emotions when they felt their goals were reaching too high, or when it seemed their ambitions would surely fail. My goal was to create a place that inspired people to be active and healthy, and to spread hope that you can reach your goals. My blog helped me along the rest of my journey as well by giving me an online community for support and encouragement during the everyday struggles of losing weight while on a college campus. I realized that although many of us have different methods for weight loss, like different eating styles and different workout preferences, we are all on the same journey together. I never dreamed my blog would blossom to the magnitude it has. I never imagined being approached in random places like shopping centers and grocery stores to have my picture taken!

I set out to create an outlet for positivity and healthy weight-loss motivation, and I accomplished more than I ever could have dreamed. Every person I interact with has an amazing story about how my blog helped them unearth their inner "fit girl." My blog has given many people the optimism they needed to believe that a big girl could be small one day. I have never claimed to have all the answers or be an expert on weight loss. Heck, at the time my blog was created, I was just a college student trying to earn decent grades in order to graduate! But my blog has become a beacon of hope bigger than me . . . and bigger than my story.

People lose weight all the time and share their stories. So what made my blog different or special? I don't know, to be honest. I don't know why my blog flourished with such force. But if I had to guess, I have a sense that it has to do with my fundamental ideas of self-love, responsibility, and inspiration. These are the core values that I emphasize on a daily basis. They are the root of my personal weight-loss philosophy, the ideas that are ingrained in almost every aspect of my personal posts and the questions I answer.

Self-Love: If you cannot love yourself at your heaviest weight, you will not love yourself at your lowest weight. This is a hard concept for people to grasp because outward beauty is something we associate with love and "perfection." And this idea of "When you're skinny, you're perfect" feeds into the delusion of skinny paving the way to self-love. The only pathway to self-love is to make the choice to love yourself. There is no number on a scale or clothing size that can make you love yourself. You have to make that conscious effort. If you wait to love yourself until you reach your goal weight . . . you will never get there. Self-love is *the* most important skill to acquire in order to have a successful weight-loss story. Don't tear down your best friend—yourself—in hopes that it will motivate you to complete your journey. Weight loss does not work that way. *Hate will never lead to a life of happiness, and self-destruction will never lead you to your goals.* Love yourself and you will always be ready to take on whatever challenges Mt. Weight Loss has in store for you. And trust me, you will face more than one challenge. But with the right skills, you will not be deterred from reaching your goals.

Like most skills, those required for having a successful weight-loss story don't come naturally. And sadly, self-love is one of those skills that doesn't come easily to people. The thought of their naked reflection in the mirror repulses them. When they see pictures of themselves, tears form in their eyes. It's okay to be upset with your weight and the habits that have taken over your life, but never for one second let those things make you think less of yourself. You are fearfully and wonderfully made, as my mom would always tell me. I never perpetually felt ugly, but there were times when I would cry and pray to God to be skinny. There were times I was upset that he made everyone else in my family small except for me. All of my friends were tiny and gorgeous . . . and all I had was a pretty face. I didn't hate myself, but I was not my number-one supporter either. I contemplated extreme calorie restriction at times. There were times when I felt so low that I thought about how much easier it would be if I just had an eating disorder. This sounds terrible, and it is terrible. But these are thoughts that the majority of people who struggle with their weight endure on a daily basis! This is self-bashing hate talk. And why?! Because you're fat. You're overweight. You're bigger than your friends and take up more space. It's ridiculous and tragic. But it's true. Those thoughts are always present. And with those thoughts comes the idea, "I will love myself when I am thin."

But self-love doesn't work that way. If you wait to love yourself it will never come. The only way to reach self-love is to choose it now.

You will not succeed on your journey if self-love is the carrot dangling at the end of the motivational string. "I can't wait to be skinny so I can love myself" is an adult fairy tale. Self-love at the end of a journey is like a maid-turned-princess at the end of a movie. It sounds great! It sounds practical! It sounds like a good, wholesome story . . . but it's unrealistic. It's right up there with the unicorns waiting for you at the top of the mountain. You have to love yourself *now*, not later.

There is no procrastination to the art of self-love. Your growth toward your goal of a healthy and happy life will not begin until you make the daily conscious effort to love yourself. Self-love is not something you can wait to accomplish, like waiting until the last minute to complete a ten-page college research paper. Self-love is not a skill developed overnight. It's a continually practiced, utilized, and evolving skill. Work on it. Cherish yourself. Love yourself. And speak kindly about your body. It's the only body you have. I would not be the person I am today without 256-pound Sharee deciding that she loved herself enough to change. You will not become the person you dream of becoming without the person you are right now. You can move, and you can change; your life does not have to be stagnant.

Responsibility: I'm a tough-love kind of person. I give tough love when I instruct fitness classes. I give tough love when I talk to people one-on-one about their goals. I give tough love when I answer questions on my blog. And I believe in tough love when it comes to taking personal responsibility for your actions. I cannot lose the weight for you. Your family, friends, co-workers, significant other, etc., cannot lose the weight for you. Only *you* can lose the weight. Only you can decide that enough is enough and that something needs to change. Your eating habits, your exercise habits, your binge-watching TV habits—all of the things preventing you from reaching your goals cannot be changed by anyone but you. Your habits created a weight problem and only you can change that.

Take responsibility for your actions and create plans that can help you reach your goals. I am all about plans! I have food schedules and menus. I grocery shop with a list. I plan and write out my workouts. I move with a purpose. You can't lollygag your way to losing a hundred pounds. You don't lose over a hundred pounds on a whim. One hundred pounds won't leave your body because you stopped drinking regular soda. It takes work, it takes effort, and it takes planning—all of which you have to take responsibility for.

I had a difficult time with this concept during the first couple years I was off at college by myself. I had terrible eating habits. I was vegan, but I still ate food like a child: processed and packaged. I refused to take responsibility over my eating habits and I halted my weight loss for almost two years. I was still active, but I was not eating responsibly. Are you eating responsibly? Planning your meals? I leave the house with all the foods I know I will need for that day: snacks, lunch, extra snacks, second lunch, etc. I am prepared! I'm prepared for if my day lasts longer than I think it will. You will get hungry, so don't leave the house without a backup food plan.

Food planning is an area where I see a lot of people lack skills. I will agree that it takes time to develop a good food-prepping system and grocery shopping regime. But just like any skill, the more you practice and develop the ability, the stronger it becomes. Food prep is now second nature to me. I don't think twice about it. Focus on developing the skills that you will need in order to be successful on your journey. Take responsibility for your food choices. Remember, no one can do it for you.

Now, some people are on the other end of food responsibility: they're so "responsible" that their eating habits have become guilt-driven, restrictive, and unhealthy. Undereating is not demonstrating responsibility. Not eating enough is just as detrimental to your health as overeating. In terms of eating, think of how you would care for a small child who is dependent on you for food sources. You are responsible for the foods that the child has access to. The only food they can eat is what you provide them. Your body is the same way! What you decide to eat is what your body gets. Eat enough! Don't starve the garden to kill the weeds. Don't be like Sarah, from Chapter 3, who thought that being healthy meant severe restriction and overexercising. Make the journey about you and take responsibility not only for your actions but also for the habits you develop along the way. Remember, those habits are what will keep you successful in terms of weight maintenance.

If you hate hitting rock bottom and starting over and over again, take the time to develop the necessary skills. It might take you a little longer to reach the top compared to those who sprint up the mountain, but what's more important? Your ability to climb up the fastest? Or your ability to maintain your goals after reaching the top? Eventually, you will no longer be in weight-loss mode and will need to make the shift to weight-management mode. It's a tough shift, so be prepared to handle it. Starvation diets are not responsible. Lack of food preparation is not responsible. Overeating is not responsible. Take responsibility to develop the behaviors required to be successful, and you *will* reach your goals.

Inspiration: Who inspires you? What inspires you? What gets you up in the morning? What is your driving force to reach your goals? If your life lacks inspiration, you won't make it far. Having aspirations and goals is great, but without inspiration, they will seem beyond your reach. Are you surrounding yourself with positivity that creates inspiration? Or are you bogged down by negative people and left feeling drained and hopeless every night when you go to bed? One of the main purposes of my blog is to serve as a place for individuals to find inspiration. I created it because all I saw online were negative individuals battling their mental illness, and that was not inspiring! It was disheartening.

Inspiration is closely related to motivation in that it has to be revisited and revamped continually. "You inspired me!" "You motivate me!" Those are two phrases I hear often on my blog, and I love it! That's what I want to do! And that's what people actually need to be searching for. What inspires you? Are you filling your life with inspiring thoughts, events, and plans that keep you positive and goal-oriented? Okay, so you might be thinking, *Yes, I need inspiration, but what does that actually look like?* And I agree, I went off on a tangent and put in a lot of words, but what does inspiration on your journey actually look like?

For me, inspiration is what helped me stay dedicated. I was inspired to be like the individuals who had lost a hundred pounds. The people in the workout DVDs I completed motivated me. The instructors in the group fitness classes I attended inspired me to do my best every single workout. Inspiration is dedication, motivation, and aspiration all rolled up into one. Without a constant investment in your inspiration funds, you will begin to lose motivation and your dedication will slip. It's hard to continually push yourself when you don't feel that urge to do so.

Think back to a time when you heard an incredible story of accomplishment. Think of how it gave you that spark of excitement. Of how instantly you began to plan your next day with a sense of anticipation and eagerness. That feeling is what you need to reestablish on a constant basis. When you stop feeling inspired, your vision of your goals will become fuzzy. A lack of inspiration leads to the opportunity for doubt, fear, and a sense of inadequacy to fill your brain. You begin to fear the unknown: What will happen when you reach your goal? Will you be happy with your new body? Will loose skin haunt you? Irrational fears and thoughts about situations that you have zero control over start to make you feel helpless and out of control. Fear will prevent you from moving forward. It's a debilitating sensation. It's normal to sense fear at some point on your journey—change is scary, especially a dramatic change such as losing weight and completely altering your daily eating and exercise habits! But it's important to not let that fear control you. You cannot control the unknown. So don't let the fear of the unknown control you. Focus on what you can control: your eating habits, your daily life choices, and your attitude—you have 100 percent control over those areas. Worrying about the unknown will leave you feeling tired, helpless, and anxious.

Another feeling that can overwhelm you when your inspiration is low is doubt. Can you reach your goal? Are you good enough to stick with it? What if you can't do everything right? What if you're wrong about your food and exercise choices? Self-doubt will paralyze you. Doubt will haunt every daily choice you make and action you take.

It will creep into every thought you have if you let it. But self-doubt is something that can be overcome when you plan for success and when you feel inspired. Do doubts happen? Yes, occasionally. But you don't need to drown in them. I found myself doubting my exercise routines. Was I doing enough? Were they the right exercises for my body? I questioned if I was giving my all when I exercised. If I didn't feel sore the next day I doubted if I had worked hard enough. Doubts will halt your progress. They will make you second-guess every choice you make. You can't doubt the process. The process works. Healthy eating and daily activity work! If your goals, healthy eating habits, and exercise routines are focused on your personal preferences, the process will work. Doubts will come and go, but like all the negative feelings you will naturally experience at times in life, you don't need to dwell in them.

A lack of inspiration can also lead to a sense of inadequacy. You will begin to question if you even deserve to be happy. Do you deserve to reach your goals? You will find yourself questioning if you're good enough. Yes, you are! You deserve to be healthy and happy. You deserve to radiate self-confidence and self-love. But when you lack inspiration, those feelings will creep in. Search for that inspiration. Seek out the stories that elicit the "I can accomplish this too" feelings. Find those individuals who accomplished what you want to accomplish. Pick their brains. Read their daily struggles. Create friendships with individuals who have similar goals and struggles.

Inspiration does not have to come from people who have already reached their goals. I have found plenty of inspiration from those still on their journey. Their continued drive to reach their goals has motivated me on days when I feel drained and worn-down. I've felt inspired by the patrons attending my fitness classes! Their intensity and focus in class have left me feeling energized and restored. You need to regularly seek that burst and rush you sense when you're inspired by someone. Find stories and build relationships with people who make you *want* to try to be the best and reach for the moon. This will give you the positivity you need on a daily basis to reach your goals.

Invest in your inspiration fund. Update your motivation board. You will not always feel passionate about a workout or feel a rush of joy ordering sweet-potato fries over onion rings. Because let's be real, onion rings are *delicious*! But those small choices and small steps you take add up. And the more inspirational relationships and stories you surround yourself with, the easier those "tough" choices and days will be. I've been there—the days when all I wanted to do was eat cake and chips—but that's not how my new healthy life works. I can't eat cake and chips all day. I can have treats, but not on an all-day, everyday basis. Remember that slippery slope of moderation mentioned earlier on? Yeah, I can't do all-day treats, because this will become a whole week of having treats. But I feel better when I eat healthier anyway! The inspirational stories I read on a daily basis and the inspirational people I surround myself with, like my mom, keep me going on those days when I just want to bury my face in a bowl of candy.

Self-love, responsibility, and inspiration are the three central focuses of my blog. My blog has helped people on their low days and it has helped me when I feel down and tired too. But social media has its downsides. When you open yourself up to the online world, this does not come without the haters. And I have a lot of haters who would love to see me fail. Initially, I was shocked to see how many individuals would go out of their way to speak ill of me. These were complete strangers, people who had zero personal interaction with me, and reacted to me based only on what they saw through pictures, posts, and online videos. It's disheartening to see random strangers hurl insults at you, from questioning your mental stability (insinuating an eating disorder) to criticizing the shape of your body. I even had people dislike my taste in clothes and bash me on social media for a jacket and shirt combo I posted.

At first, it stung! I wasn't used to that kind of negative attention. I was simply sharing my story to help inspire and motivate people, and people took it upon themselves to try to tear me down. Every ounce of me wanted to retaliate against those who attempted to hurt me. But when I took a step back and looked at the situation in a calmer frame of mind, I understood that I could grow from this. There will always be doubters, people who can't handle your positivity, people who dislike you for whatever reason. It doesn't matter how fit, happy, positive, or kind you are.

There will always be people in your life who wish you ill and want to see you fail and get hurt. But that doesn't mean you have to give in to their demands. I learned that it doesn't matter what other people think of me. If people don't believe in you, show them the person you are! People will doubt you until you prove them wrong. But also keep in mind that you don't owe anyone an explanation, ever. Let people doubt you. That has nothing to do with you! I don't care if people want to call my dedication to my goals and health "obsessive." I'm not going to apologize for completely transforming my life and sharing my story with others. Not everyone will have the same goals as you. Your dedication to completely change your life and alter your eating habits will seem odd to some people. And that's okay. What matters is that you don't let their lack of goals prevent you from wanting to reach yours. If you want to have an amazing story to tell, you have to be willing to make extraordinary changes.

If I gave in to the negativity on my blog, I would not have reached my goals. My blog continues to be a place of positivity, but there will be those individuals who attempt to make it negative. Let them. It doesn't stop me. But don't let other people's attempts to be negative in your life stop you from choosing positivity. This is your journey, your healthy life. Make it about you. Chase your dreams and create the healthy you who you've always dreamed about. You can do it.

There will be times of hardship and there will be days when you want to give up. I can't pretend that I didn't face those, because I had plenty of them! But no day ever felt as low as when I hit rock bottom. You don't ever have to feel that low again. If you're at rock bottom right now, this is the lowest you will feel. You can only go up from where you are right now. Bad days, good days, lazy days, emotional days, and stressful days, you will experience them all. It's all part of the journey. Mt. Weight Loss might not be the biggest accomplishment in your life, but it might be the focal point for a while. Creating the new healthy you will take time, and it won't happen overnight. But it will happen if you remain dedicated, consistent, and focused on making the journey about you.

My biggest accomplishment was not losing 121 pounds; it was completely transforming my life for the better. It was finally deciding that my health was worth it. And while on that journey, I found and married the love of my life, I completed my bachelor's and my master's degrees, and I created a healthy life I enjoy. You can create the healthy life you've always wanted. You can overcome Mt. Weight Loss, and if you focus on developing healthy habits along the way, the mountain range of Weight Maintenance will be something to look forward to.

Take time to reflect on the three important areas I've identified: Self-Love, Responsibility, and Inspiration. Then complete the section below.

SELF-LOVE:

Do you love yourself right now or are you waiting until you reach your goals?

____

____

____

Is your self-love approach beneficial to your journey? Are you helping or hindering your progress?

____

____

____

RESPONSIBILITY:

Are you taking responsibility for your unhealthy eating habits?

____

____

____

Are you making responsible eating choices (i.e., eating enough, eating to reach your goals, making healthy food choices, etc.)?

____

____

____

Are you eating like an adult?

____

____

____

Are you taking ownership of your weight loss and your goals?

____

____

____

INSPIRATION:

Who/what is your current inspiration?

Are you seeking out inspiration-fund fillers?

Are your sources of inspiration healthy and obtainable (i.e., unlike the sites promoting 250–calorie-a-day diets, severe food restriction, and calorie deprivation)?

Are you letting fear, self-doubt, and a sense of inadequacy prevent you from dedicating 100 percent to your goals? And if so, how can you overcome them?

12

Getting Started

We're nearing the end of the book and now you are feeling *pumped*. You have decided that enough is enough, and that it's time to get on this fitness movement, get the work done, and lose weight! But now what? Where do you start? What exercises do what? Should I do muscle building or cardio? What do I eat? Do I limit bread—can I even eat bread? Are carbs good or bad? I've shared my story and now you're ready to start writing your own story . . . but my story is not a guide. Keep in mind that no one starts the race knowing all the answers. The person on top of Mt. Weight Loss did not fall there.

Anyone who has ever successfully lost weight woke up one day with the same intentions as you. They were ready to get started and reach their goals while standing at the bottom of Mt. Weight Loss, standing there with multiple pathway options available and feeling overwhelmed about which one would get them successfully to the top.

I will not give you a meal plan to follow. We've already discussed how you need to make this journey about you and not simply copy what I did. But I would like to share some final pieces of advice to help you get started on creating your own healthy life.

Step One: Set Both Long-Term and Short-Term Goals

Short-Term Examples:

- Losing five to ten pounds
- Running a mile in under ten minutes
- Buying a piece of clothing one or two sizes too small and being able to fit into it
- Being able to do more push-ups/squats/lunges/jump roping/ jumping jacks/ burpees/etc. in one minute
- Surviving a sweets-free one-month challenge (This can be a fun way to show that you can beat your cravings.)

Long-Term Examples:

- Reaching your goal weight
- Running a marathon
- Competing in a strength or fitness challenge
- Completing an extreme obstacle course race
- Fitting into your dream size
- Wearing that outfit you've always wanted to wear that's been collecting dust in your closet for years

By setting both long-term and short-term goals you allow yourself to enjoy the journey and not just stay focused on the faraway dream. Little successes will help you see that your goals are achievable and that you can do anything you set your mind to.

Take this time to create some short-term goals and some long-term goals.

My short-term goals are:

____

____

____

My long-term goals are:

____

____

____

Step Two: Understand Your Eating Habits

I am not saying that you need to become the most nutritionally educated person and be able to write a book about the dos and don'ts of food. Step two is about understanding your eating habits and how they are either helping or hindering the goals you set for yourself in step one. Write out the eating habits that I had you identify in Chapter 4 in the space provided below.

____

____

____

Habits like this will stop you in your tracks before you even have a chance to start! Wherever you are in your journey, whether it be just starting out, halfway there, rock bottom, or wherever, take some time to identify your unhealthy eating habits. And if you don't know what unhealthy food habits you have, keep an honest food log for a few days and see what your food habits look like. Pay attention to the time of day you eat and what types of food you're eating. What time of day are you reaching for sugar? When do you crave heavy, cheesy pastas? How many "splurges" are you allowing yourself to make? Do you frequent the drive-through more often than you thought? Maybe you will see that you don't have any healthy eating habits and that all your habits are preventing you from reaching your goals. Whatever the case may be, it's always excellent to be able to honestly evaluate your habits and how they are impacting your life.

When you gain insight into your eating habits, it will help you identify what behaviors need to be replaced to help you be successful. From my experience, I see four common types of unhealthy eaters: the overeater, the emotional eater, the picky eater, and the fast-food junkie. Here are some ideas for replacement behaviors for the majority of people who fall into these categories.

The Overeater: Sometimes you will eat simply because you have nothing else to do. You might be full but you don't want to stop because the food tastes too good. Eat slower. Drink a glass of water before a meal, during the meal, and before you go back for seconds. Water is an appetite killer. Water will help you control your compulsive need to eat. Fill up on vegetables. They make you feel full and are good for you. And if you don't like vegetables . . . well, you're an adult, so eat like one. Remember, no one can lose the weight for you, so find one vegetable you can stand and learn to eat it regularly. Over time, it will get easier, I promise. But it will take time. So plan for it. Prepare the vegetables you will need. Grocery shop accordingly. If plain water tastes gross to you (I used to not be able to drink plain water too), find some of the low-calorie powder packets you can add to water. These are not the "cleanest" of products because they're loaded with chemicals and artificial sweeteners, but they never halted my progress. Everyone starts somewhere, and if this is what it will take to get you to drink water, then so be it. I won't notify the clean-food police. Focus on you and finding what works for you and your goals.

The Emotional Eater: Happy food. Sad food. Angry food. Bored food. Anxious food. Stressed food. If you're experiencing an emotion, food is there to experience it with you. If this is you, a diary or journal can help you recognize and work through your emotions without the addition of food. Food is such a huge part of our society. It's served at weddings, funerals, birthday parties, business meetings, etc., so it can be challenging to learn that food does not equal emotional coping. By keeping a journal where you write about your emotions, you can develop habits of coping that don't involve eating. If you have the urge to buy a candy bar because you have a big test tomorrow, rather than purchase the candy bar, write about it. Write out the three W's of emotional eating:

- **Why** do you want to buy the candy bar?
- **Will** the candy bar help you prepare for the test? Will it actually help solve the problem?
- **What** else can you do to take away that anxious feeling (e.g., study, go over your notes, go for a walk to clear your mind, call a friend, etc.)?

By addressing the why, will, and what questions, you can get to the root of your emotional eating. This can help you begin to realize that you don't need food to help you experience emotions. Now this might sound silly to some of you, but if you're an emotional eater, this will be a lifesaver. This process can help you better understand yourself and develop those healthy habits that will get you to your goals. Try it out for a week and see how it goes. If it's not working for you, consider meeting with a counselor to help you develop more appropriate coping skills. Reach out for the help you need! Find support groups you can join that will help you overcome this. Although the journey should be focused on you, that does not mean you're alone. There are a lot of people traveling up Mt. Weight Loss with you. Seek them out. Help each other. Share your stories, struggles, and triumphs with others. Remember, this is your journey but you don't have to tackle it alone.

The "I Hate Healthy Food" Eater (a.k.a. The Picky Eater): We all know this person (they might even be you), to whom healthy food is the devil! Healthy food is disgusting and anything that is not dipped in ranch dressing or smothered in bread crumbs is inedible. Honestly, the healthy habit switch you need to make is to simply grow up. You're not a child. You're an adult. If this is you, you're acting the way I did when I pouted at the grocery store in Scotland because it "didn't have any food." It's ridiculous! Sometimes tough love is what it takes. If you and I were having coffee and you said, "Sharee, losing weight is hard because I just don't like anything healthy," I would look at you and kindly say, "You know what else is hard? Having type 2 diabetes at the age of forty-five. Not being able to run around with your kids because your knees hurt so much. Praying that every building has an elevator because your body can't handle a couple flights of stairs." That stuff is hard . . . eating healthy is hard only if you make it hard. *So choose your type of hard.*

I don't want to come across as mean, because I'm not. I am direct. I want you to hear how ridiculous it sounds if you're holding yourself back because of the taste of healthy food. Buy a cookbook and find some recipes that appeal to you. This is your health! Your life matters. Your goals matter. I know a bag of chips might sound better than an apple. But an apple won't clog your arteries. Living on fast food and junk . . . that is how you dig your grave with a fork, one french fry at a time. There are lifelong implications for individuals who refuse to take responsibility for their eating habits and assume an attitude of "This is too hard." I know it's hard. I've been there before. But I am telling you that *you can do this*. You can end the vicious dieting cycle.

This has nothing to do with reaching a goal weight or being skinny. This is about health. I do not believe you need to be 135 pounds to be healthy. I do believe that you need to live an active life and eat the right foods. It doesn't matter if you're 135 pounds or 275 pounds. If you would have to reconsider your survival options if you needed to run a mile . . . that's not healthy. I may hate running, but I guarantee you, if the zombie apocalypse ever happens, my body is conditioned enough to run for hours. If that isn't motivation, I don't know what is!

The Fast-Food Survivalist: Your survival in life depends on access to fast-food chains. Breakfast is routinely consumed in your car after a stop at your favorite drive-through. Lunch is always combo number two, the workers know your order by heart, and 99 percent of the time your order is ready before you even arrive. And takeout dinner is so routine that you have a tab at the restaurant. You live on fast food, and when it's not ordered at a drive-through you're eating out of a package from the grocery store's snack aisle. Now some people reading this might be laughing because it's so foreign to them. But others will relate to it on some level. The idea of prepping food and bringing a lunch to work is only a myth to some. Well, I'm here to tell you that it's not a myth. And *if* you want to reach your goals, you're going to need to stop reaching for your wallet at a drive-through and start reaching for plastic food-storage containers and a lunch box.

You are going to get hungry at work, at school, while out shopping, and while running errands. So pack your food! Prepare your meals. You won't eat unhealthy junk foods if you're too busy filling up on healthy foods. Making a lunch is not rocket science. It takes two minutes to put together a peanut butter sandwich and cut up an apple. And if that doesn't sound appealing to you, how does having a heart attack at the age of forty sound? How does being overweight for your entire life sound? How do achy joints, bad knees, and type 2 diabetes sound? You might be okay health-wise right this moment, but keep going down that path and your choices will catch up to you. You can't outrun a bad diet. Your body eventually will reflect on the outside the abuse you ingested over the years. I have included a meal idea section in the last chapter of the book. Give it some thought! You can do this! It will take time and effort, but it is completely within your realm of control.

And one more thing before I move on: don't eat fast food. Just stop. Stop lying to yourself and be honest about what you're putting into your body. Fast food is not real food. Remember, eat for your goals. Healthy, active goal-reachers—at least this one—do not eat fast food. It's a terrible habit that is ravaging this nation. Fruits can be grabbed faster than a burger can be made. And if your excuse is "Healthy food doesn't taste as good," then you're simply not applying yourself in the kitchen. Healthy food can taste wonderful! Read the picky eater section again and take notes. You need to overcome the fast-food habit, because your health depends on it. You can live off fast-food products for only so long. Eventually, your body will say, "Enough is enough," and I pray that you're able to recover from the severity of that wake-up call.

Step Three: Clean Up Your Eating

So you figured out where you're messing up. You might not relate 100 percent to the scenarios that I listed above, but maybe you can relate on some level. Here are some additional tips to help you replace your current goal-stoppers with goal-reaching behaviors. I have created an easy-to-follow five-week clean-eating challenge that can help you focus on taking the little steps that will lead to big changes.

Week 1: Add a Serving of Fruits or Vegetables to Every Meal: By adding fruits and veggies to every meal, you will not only fill up faster but also learn that veggies and fruits are yummy and not hard to eat. The nutrients from fruits and veggies are hard to find in processed foods. Your body needs and craves the real stuff. Here are some suggestions and tips.

- If you are making a peanut butter and jelly sandwich use fruit instead of jelly! Strawberry slices are delicious and fresh. The crunch from an apple is one of my favorite combinations with peanut butter. Banana with peanut butter is also a classic combination. Peanut butter and raspberry—delicious! The goal is to add fruit in any way you can.
- Wraps are an excellent way to add vegetables into your day. I have a few ideas in the last chapter of the book. Use your favorite salad dressing or spread (my personal favorite is hummus) as the base of the wrap and load up with vegetables. You can use raw or cooked vegetables: mushrooms, green peppers, cucumbers, carrots, lettuce, spinach, celery, olives, beans, tomatoes, squash, zucchini, broccoli—there is no limit. Get creative. Find a combination you love! Also, don't be shy to add some protein. Walnuts pair great with pear slices, spinach, and mustard for us vegans. Or if you eat meat, try a spicy chicken wrap with salsa, black beans, shredded

carrots, spinach, and sautéed mushrooms. Healthy does not have to be boring.
- Swap a bag of chips for a cup of grapes or blueberries. Or for an extra-sweet treat, try eating frozen grapes. They taste amazing!

Week 2: No More Fast Food—Ever! We already addressed this issue, but just in case it wasn't clear the first time: STOP. EATING. FAST. FOOD. Fast food is damaging. It has nothing real in it. Regardless of the ads on TV, use your brain. It's awful. Think of your favorite fitness idol . . . or favorite Hollywood celebrity trainer. Do you see them eating fast food? Remember, eat for your goals.

But what about treat or "cheat" meals? Well, I prefer to use the term "treat" meal myself, and yes, I support the idea of having a treat meal every week. But if I'm going to treat myself, it's not going to be on some fake food. I'm going to have an epic treat of *real* food. So just keep that in mind. What do you want to put in your body? Fake food or real food? Also keep in mind whether moderation is something that you are not able to do at this time. When you schedule your treats—and do make sure they're scheduled and not just a spur-of-the-moment type of thing—plan to eat at a restaurant or another place where the food is controlled for you. The worst thing you could possibly do is go to the grocery store and buy your treats. There is zero structure and absolutely zero accountability. You will walk out of the store with five bags of candy and enough chips to feed a small army. This is a treat meal, not a treat to send you to your grave.

Week 3: Switch to Wheat or Brown Bread, Pasta, and Rice: Whole grain is healthy and also more filling for you! It's full of fiber and everything healthy that is sucked out of white bread, pasta, and rice. Eat it. Restaurants and cafeterias typically offer this option; you just need to ask for it. If you're unsure about the taste, try half white and half wheat and slowly increase the wheat ratio. Calorie-wise, wheat products and white products are pretty similar. This is not about calories, though, it's about nutrition and the quality of your nutrition. Whole-wheat products provide higher nutritional values than their white-product counterparts. Calories are not created equally; it's what makes up those calories that counts. And wheat is the champion in this case.

Week 4: Base Every Snack on a Fruit or Veggie: This will teach you that fruits and veggies can be more than just side dishes; they can be eaten during the day when those snack cravings hit.

Here are some healthy snack options (more are included in the last chapter):

- Apples with peanut butter
- Strawberries with Cool Whip
- Vegetables with hummus
- Peaches with cottage cheese
- Yogurt with fruit
- Sliced or balled melons
- Frozen grapes or blueberries
- Fresh fruit smoothies (one cup liquid base, one frozen banana, one cup of frozen berries)
- Bananas with peanut butter
- Celery sticks with seasoning salt or peanut butter
- Cucumbers with hummus or pesto

Week 5: No More Soda: The amount of sugar in one can of soda is mind-blowing. You will never reach your goals unless you break up with soda and juice. There is a better liquid out there for you called water. Water will love you! And your body loves water! It's practically made of water! I know water is not the most exciting thing in the world, but we are talking about your health and your goals. Water will help you reach them!

No more soda. What helps me feel motivated to drink water is carrying around a cute water bottle with me wherever I go. It keeps my hands busy and gives me something to do rather than reach for food. Water is your friend, so embrace it. And as mentioned previously in this chapter, you can add flavored powder packets to your water until you get used to drinking it. Try a one-to-one ratio: for every flavored water you drink you have to drink a glass of plain water. There is no substitute for water. It's essential for our bodies' survival. But I know it takes time to develop the healthy habit of chugging water. Give it time, and just like all the other healthy habits you're going to focus on developing, your ability to drink water will gradually strengthen.

Step Four: Find Your Fitness Style

Not everyone was made to be a runner. I mentioned earlier, the thought of running makes me want to never leave my house. But I love Zumba, boot camp–style classes, and total body conditioning classes. I like being around people and sweating until there are puddles. But I can't run to save my life . . . It's too boring for me. And that is okay. There are tons of fitness options out there! Set yourself up for success by picking an activity you will learn to love (it takes time, but it will happen), and also pick a time that will work for you. I can't work out at 5:00 a.m. . . . ever. I would fail at reaching my goals if that were the only time I dedicated to my fitness. So pick a time that will work for you and pick a type of fitness that will work for you! Create a healthy, fit life you will enjoy, not a life full of restrictions and constant body-bashing. Exercise is not punishment; it's a method for improving quality of life. Enjoy it, and you will enjoy your life.

Here are some fitness ideas:

- Women's-only gym
- Personal training
- Group training (semi-private personal training)
- Gym with options you would utilize
- Group fitness classes
- Fitness apps on your phone
- In-home DVD programs (with all those commercials that come on at night promoting a fitness program, I'm sure there is one that has caught your attention; give it a try!)
- Stationary cycling
- Joining a cycling group, walking club, or running group

Step Five: Create Your Goal Board

All the hard work you put into creating the perfect plan to help you reach your goals deserves to be hung up! So create a board with your goals on display, both your short-term and long-term goals. Type up the five-week clean-eating challenge and hang it up. Create a calendar to keep you organized. Place a sticker on your planned treat days. Have your gym's group fitness schedule in sight so you always know what "meetings" you have for the week. Hang up motivational quotes and transformation pictures. Have a designated "quote of the week," something that speaks to your current mood and feelings. Display things that will help you remain dedicated. Motivation will come and go; dedication is what will drive you to get results. Create your goal board and you will be on your way to creating the fit-and-healthy you.

So there you have it. That is as "guided" as I will get because this is about *you* and your journey, not what I did on mine. My story shows that success is possible, and that you can create the healthy life you've always wanted and be the person you daydream about. Take charge. Get active. And wear black for your own funeral for your fat.

13

Grocery List and Meal Ideas

Although my book is not a guide, I felt it would be important to include some ideas for a grocery list, to help provide a simple starting place for those who are overwhelmed with the thought of doing a pantry and fridge overhaul. I also thought it would be supportive and helpful to share some simple meal and snack ideas. Again, this is your journey, so make it about you! But I hope my ideas will help you get moving in the right direction.

The meal ideas are suggestions, so please take into account your own individual calorie and dietary needs. Not eating enough of the right things is just as bad as overeating. Both can impact your weight and health in a negative way. Find what works for you! I have also included ideas for my non-veg-head readers. I don't want anyone to feel left out—just because going vegan worked for me does not mean it will work for you! So find what works for you and run with it. Make your journey enjoyable. Most importantly, make it a genuine reflection of you.

Grocery List Example

FRUITS:

- Apples
- Pears
- Bananas
- Berries: raspberries, strawberries, blueberries (can be purchased frozen for smoothies)
- Melons: watermelon, cantaloupe
- Grapes
- Cherries (frozen works great for smoothies)
- Mandarin oranges
- Plums
- Peaches
- Nectarines

PROTEIN:

- Meat alternatives: tofu, seitan, tempeh, veggie burgers (look for brands that include real vegetables in the patties)
- Lean meats: chicken breast, turkey
- Nut butters: peanut, almond (my personal favorites)
- Protein powder (if you find yourself wanting some)
- Eggs

VEGETABLES:

- Tomatoes
- Broccoli
- Green beans
- Carrot sticks
- Celery
- Peppers: green, red, yellow
- Asparagus
- Squash
- Mushrooms
- Zucchini
- Lettuce (bagged veggie blend)
- Canned kidney beans and corn (low sodium)
- Stewed tomatoes
- Snap peas
- Bean sprouts
- Cauliflower
- Potatoes
- Onions: red, yellow, green

CARBS: (Yes, you can eat carbs!)

- Whole-wheat bread
- Whole-wheat tortilla wraps
- Oatmeal
- Granola
- Whole-grain cereal
- Brown rice
- Pita bread
- English muffins (I love whole grain and cinnamon raisin)

DAIRY:

- Milk alternatives: soy, almond, rice, cashew
- Milk: skim, low fat
- Cheese: skim, low fat
- Yogurt: Greek, regular, coconut, almond, soy (low-sugar and high-protein options recommended)

SNACKS:

- Mixed nuts (pre-packaged to avoid oversnacking)
- Hummus
- Whole-grain crackers
- Dried fruit (no-sugar-added)
- Protein and/or granola bars (a one-to-one ratio for protein and sugar recommended)

OTHER:

- Peanut butter (on the list twice because it's amazing!)
- Salad dressing (check sodium content)
- Sweet-and-sour sauce
- Low-sodium soy sauce
- Hemp seeds
- Canned soup (low sodium)
- Low-sodium canned chili (making your own is always fun too)
- Shredded coconut
- Slivered or crushed nuts: walnuts, almonds, peanuts (great salad toppers)

Meal Ideas

BREAKFAST

- Oatmeal bowls:
  - Blueberry and Peanut Butter Oats: oatmeal, blueberries, peanut butter, chopped almonds, cinnamon (I use frozen blueberries and cook them with the oats; it makes them more gooey.)
  - Apple Pie Oats: oatmeal, diced apples, cinnamon, chopped walnuts, peanut butter (The peanut butter is optional, but you just can't go wrong with peanut butter!)
  - Berry Goodness Oats: oatmeal, sliced bananas, raspberries, blueberries, hemp seeds, peanut butter (If you cook the bananas with the oats, they become gooey-yummy-goodness.)
  - Chocolate and Peanut Butter Oats: oatmeal, sliced bananas, cocoa powder, crunchy peanut butter, shredded coconut

- Whole-grain cereal with fruit slices
- Yogurt topped with granola and fresh fruit slices
- Whole-wheat peanut butter toast with banana slices

SMOOTHIES:

- Peanut Butter Espresso: frozen banana, peanut butter, cocoa powder, milk of choice, shots of espresso (I like vanilla almond milk or vanilla soy milk.)
- PB & J: frozen banana, frozen strawberries, peanut butter, milk of choice
- Tropical Delight: frozen banana, frozen mango slices, frozen pineapple chunks, shredded coconut, milk of choice (You can top this with additional shredded coconut.)
- Cherry Madness: frozen banana, frozen cherries, vanilla yogurt of choice, cocoa powder, milk of choice
- Mixed Berry Bliss: frozen banana, frozen blueberries, frozen raspberries, frozen strawberries, milk of choice

MID-MORNING SNACK:

- Apple slices with peanut butter
- Carrot and celery sticks with hummus topped with hemp seeds
- Protein and/or granola bar with a banana
- Latte with mixed nuts (I'm a coffee junkie, so I frequent coffee shops on a regular basis. Coffee is how I made it through eight years of college!)
- Frozen grapes and blueberries with yogurt

LUNCH:

- Loaded salads (add chicken or omit as desired):
  - Bean Salad: kidney beans, black beans, garbanzo beans, chopped green onions, shredded carrots, sliced olives, grape tomatoes, sliced avocado, lettuce, topped with freshly squeezed lemon and hummus
  - Chicken Salad: shredded baked chicken, chopped walnuts, dried cranberries, shredded carrots, hemp seeds all on a bed of lettuce dressed with fruit vinaigrette dressing or light dressing of choice

- Mexi-Flare Salad: cooked brown rice, black beans, corn, shredded carrots, chopped cilantro, olives, sliced green and red peppers (cooked or raw), lettuce, topped with your favorite salsa (This also makes a delicious wrap!)
- Loaded Salad: chopped apples, diced cucumbers, chopped pears, kidney beans, slivered almonds, corn, lettuce, topped with dressing of choice

- Wrap with whole-wheat tortilla:
  - Hummus and Vegetable: mushrooms (cooked or raw), peppers, onions, zucchini, olives, lettuce, hummus
  - Sweet Chicken: baked chicken, sliced pears, walnut halves, dried cranberries or cherries, romaine lettuce, Dijon mustard
  - Crunchy Veggie: shredded carrots, romaine lettuce, cucumber slices, zucchini, walnut halves, Dijon and yellow mustard combo as spread
- Peanut butter whole-wheat sandwich topped with sliced apples served with carrot sticks and hummus
- Soup (low sodium) with whole-wheat crackers or toast
- Toasted English muffin topped with poached or scrambled egg served with fruit

MID-DAY SNACK:

- Homemade trail mix: mixed nuts, shredded coconut, dried fruit (no sugar added)
- Protein bar or granola bar with fruit slices
- Peanut butter toast or toasted English muffin with peanut butter
- Protein smoothie (options from breakfast but with protein powder in place of peanut butter)
- Carrot sticks with mixed nuts or peanut butter
- Cucumber slices with seasoning salt

DINNER:

- Whole-wheat pasta with grilled veggies topped with red pasta sauce (To add some extra protein, add baked chicken or a vegan meat alternative.)
- Sautéed vegetables (mushrooms, peppers, zucchini, squash) served with pita bread and hummus

- Healthy pizza: Top an English muffin with toppings of choice, such as pasta sauce, veggies, healthy cheese options, and chicken or a meat alternative. Toast in the oven at 350 degrees for seven to ten minutes. Serve with steamed broccoli, corn, and cauliflower.
- Loaded salad from the lunch options
- Wrap from the lunch options

SWEET TREAT*:

- Quick "baked" apples: Top thinly sliced apples with cinnamon, an alternative sweetener of choice (Splenda, Truvia, Stevia, agave nectar, honey, etc.) and chopped almonds. Microwave for two minutes and thirty seconds. Add peanut butter if you want some warm sauce on top. (It's like apple pie but without the calories!)
- Peanut butter toast topped with strawberry slices and shredded coconut
- Smoothie crunch bowl: Any of the smoothies listed under the breakfast options can be made thicker and more sorbet-like by reducing the liquid content (i.e., rather than one cup of milk, add two tablespoons of milk and water until desired consistency is reached). Top with granola chunks. Get your ice cream fix.
- Protein-packed "cookie": Heat up a protein bar in the microwave. It's like a gooey cookie packed with protein.
- Raw apple slices drizzled with melted peanut butter

*Dessert has a bad reputation in the fad-diet culture. How many friends do you know who follow the "no food after 7:00 p.m." rule? Honestly, I've always been a late-night eater. Between teaching fitness classes until 9:00 p.m. and working on homework until obscene hours of the night, I *had* to eat late. I didn't have a choice. The thing is, calories can't tell time. What does matter is what you eat. Reach for healthy foods and your body will reward you. Most people reach for junk food at night and that is why they experience weight gain. It has more to do with what people are eating late at night, not when they eat. Healthy food will change your life.

Items to Avoid When Shopping:

Processed Deli Meats: Processed meats are typically high in sodium and chemical fillers. Look for low-sodium and all-natural options. Or purchase freshly sliced lean meats from the deli counter at your local grocery store. Sodium is not something your body needs any extra of.

If meat is something you are going to include in your journey, that is your choice. Deli meats are great for quick sandwiches, wraps, and salads. You just want to make sure that you're purchasing the right kinds of meats. Processed meats are not the same as fresh or all-natural meats. Always check ingredient lists or purchase freshly cut meats that don't need a label. Your health is important and so are your goals. Shop smart and shop healthfully.

Baked Goods: Cookies, pies, cakes, cupcakes, muffins, etc.—these items are loaded with sugar, fat, sodium, and calories, nothing your body needs and nothing that will help you reach your goals. A standard-sized muffin can easily pack over four hundred calories! Even "natural" and "organic" baked goods are loaded with sugar and fat. A cookie is a cookie. Avoid buying processed baked goods and stick to the natural sugars that are found in fruit. Fruit is loaded with tons of great vitamins and minerals. And although it's full of sugar, fruit has fiber. And fiber is the difference between ingesting a tablespoon of white sugar and eating an apple. Whole fruit (including the skin) is so good for you. Fruit will not make you fat. But it does have calories, so you want to watch your overall caloric intake to ensure you're eating for your goals. But fruit is healthy and good for you and should be included in your daily life.

What's a good alternative when a baked-good desire strikes? Homemade breakfast "cookies" fulfill my cookie sweet tooth. I use the word "cookie" lightly, as these are basically baked oatmeal rolled into cookie-sized balls. All I do is mash up a ripe banana in a bowl, add about a three-quarter cup of oats, some vanilla, some chopped nuts, a splash of almond or soy milk, and add some frozen blueberries. I mix everything up, roll the mixture into cookie-sized balls, place them on a baking sheet, and bake them in the oven for about ten to twelve minutes.

The result is a soft and flavorful cookie-like treat that is simply my morning oatmeal bowl prepared in a different way. And the best thing is that you can combine different types of ingredients to suit your taste buds. The base of these "cookies" is the banana and oats; the rest is whatever you want. Shredded coconut, chopped cherries, raspberries, chocolate chips, cocoa powder, peanut butter, etc.—the possibilities are endless. And what is great about this "cookie" recipe is that it won't halt your progress. You get the best of both worlds. Healthy can be exciting and flavorful. And if anyone tries to tell you that healthy is boring, they simply aren't doing it right.

Chips and Crackers: Salty and crunchy is my favorite combination. Add chocolate and we've got a home run. But when it comes to reaching your goals, chips and crackers tend to be people's pitfall foods. They are for me, at least. I could eat a whole bag of tortilla chips in one sitting if given the opportunity. So not only are these unhealthy foods, they are also difficult to practice portion control with. Who wants to eat only twelve chips? Not me. So chips and crackers are on my "Items to Avoid" list for the simple fact that they pack hidden calories and are difficult to control portion-wise. Whole-wheat crackers can be a healthy alternative, but ensure that you aren't tempted to eat the whole box. Healthy food calories matter too.

When I am craving something sweet, salty, and crunchy, I heat up some thinly sliced apples in the microwave and top them with peanut butter, cinnamon, and crushed mixed nuts. This delivers the perfect amount of crunch, sweetness, and saltiness, but without stopping me from reaching my goals. It's all about finding healthy ways to eat, not depriving yourself. It's about developing the skill set to fulfill your body's cravings with natural, healthy foods and not food-like products.

Cravings are the body's natural way of telling us that it's lacking sufficient nutrients of some sort, such as iron, sodium, calcium, etc. For example, if you find yourself craving carbonation, that is your body's natural way of telling you that your calcium is low.

Carbonation pulls calcium from our bones, which then allows our bodies to use it. Your body pulling calcium from your bones is not healthy! That leads to serious health complications as we age. Calcium is what keeps our bones strong and healthy. And if your body is forced to pull calcium from your bones, something is wrong.

So understanding that cravings *mean* something can help you address them in a healthy way versus in an unhealthy way. I remember a time when I had low calcium levels and all I wanted to drink were energy drinks! I remember being so surprised at this weird craving I was having because I was well into my fitness and healthy eating regimens by that point. But I had the irresistible urge to drink energy drinks every time I completed a rigorous workout! It wasn't until I began to research the cause that I discovered my body was trying to find ways to get calcium. I began taking calcium supplements and the cravings went away.

This journey is an opportunity for you to learn about yourself and your body. Learn, study, and take time to research what works for you and what your body is trying to tell you. Research your cravings; you might find some useful and interesting information.

Soda and Juice: Soda and juice are calorie-and-sugar bombs. There are zero nutritional benefits in either product. Let's focus on soda first. Soda is nothing but carbonation, sugar syrup, and chemicals. It's literally liquid sugar crap that is a recipe for addiction. If I were in charge of labeling items realistically, this is what I would put on the labels of sodas: "Liquid Sugar Crap—The Recipe for Addiction." But for the sake of soda sales, I think soda manufacturers would frown upon that label.

The amount of sugar in soda will blow your mind. And to think that there are individuals who drink liters of soda a day is astonishing to me! You will not reach your goals if you continue to consume soda. If you continue to drink soda, the chemical reaction that drinking soda causes in your body will prevent you from overcoming your sugar addiction. I don't need a background in nutrition to know that. I've taken my fair share of physiological psychology classes to know that sugar and crack display similar chemical addiction patterns in the brain. If you want to overcome your addiction to junk food, soda is the most powerful place to start.

Diet soda, while it does not have sugar, still has the same chemicals and elicits the same chemical patterns as regular soda. I've personally noticed that drinking diet soda only makes me want more soda. I'm not a nutritionist, but I do have a story and some hefty experiences that provide some valuable insight into addiction and food. So take my diet soda advice with a grain of salt, but know that I felt a lot better when I cut soda altogether. I was in denial about diet soda and its harmfulness for a long time, but I eventually listened to my inner health nut and cut the habit. And I do feel much better.

Now let's talk about juice. If fruit is okay, why is fruit juice on my "Items to Avoid" list? Because fruit juice is not the same as whole fruit. When you take the fiber and the skin out of the fruit, all the nutrients go with them. The fiber in fruit is the best part for us! So if you're drinking just the juice . . . all the goodness has been wrung out and all you've been left with is sugar. Fiber, that's what you want.

What about the ready-made fruit smoothies you see at stores in the produce section? Well, this will come down to personal preference and what works for you. I would rather make my own smoothie so I can control the ingredients and specific amounts of what I put in it. If you like the ready-made smoothies and you're seeing progress with them included in your daily diet, then I don't see any reason to discontinue drinking them. This is about *you* and not about what worked specifically for me.

My lifestyle won't yield results for everyone. What will give results is simply being healthy and active, and that will look different based on the individual. Everyone on Mt. Weight Loss will have a different path, but ultimately everyone is going in the same direction. So it's okay to disagree with me or prefer things differently—that is life! Different points of views lead to the best conversations and opportunities to expand our own thoughts. I 100 percent accept the reality that some people reading this book disagree with me on a variety of topics. And that is okay. This is not an argument; it's a personal story with some advice thrown into the mix. It's not enforcing the rules of weight loss and providing the ultimate key to a healthy life. Find *your* path up Mt. Weight Loss. That is what is important, not who takes the same path as you.

Candy: Oh, good old candy. I love candy. But candy does not love my goals. Candy is right up there with chemical and sugar addiction. Candy is addictive. It's easy to eat a king-sized pack of candy in one sitting without even stopping to think twice about the calories. Candy is another calorie bomb. Two or three pieces can be above and beyond two hundred calories, and no one stops at just two or three pieces—not if you have a weight problem, at least. It's best to just avoid candy altogether. Kick the habit and stop purchasing it. The longer you go without candy, the less your cravings will become. Because it's sugar, you will initially face intense cravings for candy. But once you get past the initial extinction burst (when the behavior you're trying to decrease becomes incredibly intense for a brief amount of time), you will come out stronger and be that much closer to your goals of developing lasting, healthy eating habits.

Frozen Entrées: This is another area where you either agree with me or disagree with me. Some people see great results eating "healthy" ready-made frozen entrées. I am not that person. Whereas I did eat them sparingly while losing weight, they were not included in my daily eating routine. Frozen meals, even the healthy and "light" options, tend to be higher in sodium, fat, and sugar content. The calories might be in the okay range, but remember, all calories are not created equally, and when you're trying to overcome a food and sugar addiction, it's really important to pay attention to what makes up those calories. I would rather make my own whole-wheat pasta dish and be able to control the ingredients and salt content rather than use a pre-made microwavable entrée. This is an area where you will have to see what works for you and your goals.

If the ready-made light options keep you away from the deep-fried takeout you routinely order, then I would start there. But keep in mind that the target is for you to reach your goals, replace your unhealthy eating habits, and feel healthy. You can't fake being healthy and fit. The only way to achieve a healthy and fit body is to engage in activities that healthy and fit people engage in.

14

Frequently Asked Questions

Below you will find the shortened, but detailed, answers to many frequently asked questions I receive on a daily basis. If you want a quick boost of motivation and insight, or want answers on a specific topic, this can be a good place to find some useful information without having to read an entire chapter.

Losing weight is so overwhelming and I don't know where to start. How did you get started?

I know it's overwhelming. Looking an extra hundred pounds in the face is not something that sparks a sense of "I can do it!" It took me a few attempts to actually find a method that worked for me. I tried various diets and ways of eating until I stumbled on the vegan diet. And that is what clicked for me. Again, the weight did not just fall off; it took me five years. Five years to reach my goals—that is a long time. I started with small steps. I focused on food and then branched out into exercise-related fitness. Just like with food, it took me a few different attempts to find something that I enjoyed enough to keep going back to.

If you're really lost on where to start, think about the type of fit or healthy person you want to be. Do you want to be one of those guys or girls in the gym lifting weights? Do you want to be the person who wakes up early in the morning to go for a run? Do you want to be the person who takes cycling classes in the evening, followed by a boot camp class? Are you drawn to people who drink smoothies all the time and eat granola bowls regularly? What are these individuals doing? Model it. If you know the type of fit person you want to be, fake it until you make it. If you want to be like the girl who gets up and runs every morning, find a running guide for beginners and get started. If you want to be the person at the gym lifting weights, seek out the help of a personal trainer or find some online resources for beginners. You could also join a gym that has daily weight-lifting workouts that you complete in groups. Find the type of fit person you want to be and replicate their routine as a beginner. It's important that you create a regimen that matches your fitness abilities. You won't be able to perform at the same level as your sources of fitness inspiration at first, but you can create a similar training style suitable for a beginner.

If you have absolutely no idea of what type of fit person you want to be, but you just know that you want to lose weight and feel better, don't stress. Find an exercise that you're curious about trying, like a group fitness class, cycling, boot camp, an in-home workout program, etc. Try out different exercises until you find one that makes you say, "Yeah, I can stick with this for a while." Then stick with it. There is no magic remedy for weight loss. There is no one-size-fits-all plan. Finding a form of fitness you can learn to love and learning to embrace healthy foods are what it takes to create a successful weight-loss story.

Food is something that will vary depending on the individual. The most important factors regarding weight loss and food are eating enough, eating the right things, and eating responsibly. This includes taking responsibility for your eating habits and learning to replace unhealthy habits with healthy ones. You're an adult or young adult, so it's time to learn to have a bowl of fruit with some peanut butter toast for breakfast, not a fast-food burrito every morning. Eat enough food. You cannot create a healthy body eating a minimal amount of calories.

Twelve hundred calories is *not* the magic number for weight loss. You will need more.

The last concept is eating the right things. This concept will look different depending on the person. I'm vegan, which works for me. A vegan diet would not work for my husband. However, we both eat healthfully. What does healthy look like for you? The typical healthy staples are vegetables, fruits, whole grains, low-fat dairy options, lean meats and meat alternatives, seeds, nuts, etc. Foods that are typically avoided or limited in a healthy diet include processed foods and packaged foods (basically the entire snack food aisle at the grocery store), fried foods, fast foods, etc. There is a whole variety of ways to eat healthfully; you just need to find which way works for you and your body. It will take time to develop a routine, but it's not impossible. You can do it. Give it time and allow yourself to learn. You will grow and be stronger at the end of the journey. Check out Chapter 12 for additional tips.

Are you actually happy with your stretch marks?

Well, I am not exactly throwing a party to celebrate having them, but I don't hide them or feel the need to cover myself up. I can't control my stretch marks. I have absolutely zero ability to ever make them go away. No amount of creams, exercise, weight loss, light therapy, or exfoliation will make them go away. Why would I continue to focus on something that I can't control? Am I thrilled I have them? Not really. But honestly, I don't actually think about them anymore. I don't notice them because I've moved on.

When people ask me about stretch marks, I think, *Oh yeah, I do have those.* But they're removed from my mind because I spend zero time focusing on them. I was devastated when they began to develop when I was younger. I was embarrassed to change in the locker rooms in middle school. I was the only person I knew who had them. Both my mom and sister are stretch mark free, and that used to really bother me. But I can't control my stretch marks. They have since faded to a pale white, and with a good spray tan they are barely visible. My advice for "dealing" with stretch marks is that there are so many more significant and greater concerns that will arise on your weight-loss journey. Focus on what you can control, not on what you can't. Stretch marks are a part of life, not a life-altering or life-ending experience.

Check out Chapter 8 for more information on how to "deal" with stretch marks.

I feel so alone. I don't have anyone I can talk to about my weight loss and no one in my family supports me.

Starting the journey up Mt. Weight Loss is a scary endeavor. If you're alone on your journey, it's even scarier. That fear and crushing sense of loneliness can bring you plummeting back to rock bottom. Unfortunately, I don't have a simple solution. I don't have an easy-to-follow method to gain support on your journey and create lasting and meaningful friendships. It's a hard place to be mentally, physically, and emotionally. While I don't have a quick-fix remedy, I do have some tips that might help you branch out and find ways to feel supported on your journey.

Join a weight-loss program at your local gym or an online weight-loss program. Many weight-loss programs offer meeting locations in your local area. Search online to find a weight–loss-program meeting in your area. While it might take some branching out of your comfort zone, this can be a great opportunity for you to meet like-minded individuals and help create a sense of support. While you are the only person who can lose your weight, that does not mean you have to take the journey alone. There are lots of people on their journey up Mt. Weight Loss; you can make the climb together. If you can't attend a local meeting or one is not offered in your area, many weight-loss programs have online opportunities that will provide support and access to weight-loss communities too.

Online weight-loss communities, such as blogs like mine, are other places where you can connect with individuals who are chasing similar goals as you. There is a whole online world with individuals sharing their stories, daily struggles, experiences, and everyday lives while on their journey. These online communities can be a great source of motivation, support, friendship, and inspiration. Oftentimes, you can even find local people and schedule a meet-up with lots of online weight-loss community individuals. This online community can be a place where you reach out for help in specific situations. It can be an outlet for you to talk about your own struggles and seek advice from others who might have experienced similar situations. While it does not replace the support of your family and close friends, it will help you to not feel so alone.

If you don't have the support around you, build it. Find that online community to reach out to. Or maybe post something on your own social media pages. Post that you are looking for friends who would like to join a support circle. Weight loss is a common goal; lots of individuals decide at some point in time that they want to lose weight. I'm sure there are some people whom you are friends with online who want to lose weight too. Start the conversation and create a support group. If the support you want is not around you, create it. It won't be easy, but it is something that can be done. This is your journey. Embrace it and take the steps you need to be successful.

This is my first year at a university and I don't want to gain the "freshman 15." Help!

There is an unrealistic belief that when you leave for college, you automatically gain fifteen pounds. This idea is that freedom while away at school equates to unwarranted weight gain. You will not gain weight unless your actions promote it. If you eat junk, party all night, and neglect physical movement apart from walking to class and parties, you will gain weight. There is no alternative if that is how you decide your college experience will be. You don't gain weight unless your actions promote weight gain (this obviously doesn't include those with health conditions).

If you eat right, move often, and do more than drink and party, you will not gain weight. You do not need to be intoxicated every night in order to have a wonderful college experience. I don't drink. I had not even tasted alcohol until I was twenty-one years old and legally able to drink. Alcohol was never something that I wanted to participate in. In my opinion it tastes terrible, is a complete waste of calories, and provides absolutely zero nutritional benefit to my body. So I was never one who went to parties and drank the night away. However, I do know that for some people, partying is something they deem as imperative while away at college. There is this idea that it's not truly a college experience until you can't remember half the nights you spent there.

Here's my opinion: be an adult. Eat with a purpose. Venture to the student gym. You will gain weight if you don't take actions to be healthy. You will be stressed because of schoolwork, and if you don't have established healthy-eating habits, you will reach for chips, candy, cookies, soda, and pizza. Even though I was on my healthy journey in college, I still fell victim to late-night stress-eating cycles. Stress will hit you and you will want to eat. Having healthy eating habits can turn those moments into healthy snack moments versus emergency fast-food hauls. You can't control the amount of schoolwork and exams thrown at you, but you can control the foods you eat, the exercise you participate in, and the healthy habits you strive to create.

For more information on managing stress and school life, check out Chapter 10.

Are you embarrassed about your tummy-tuck scar?

I was once a size twenty-two/twenty-four and 256 pounds. I had a doctor tell me that I would never be small, and now I wear a size two/four. I went from being unable to complete a push-up or a mile-long run without feeling like my lungs were going to catch on fire, to teaching fitness classes and sharing my weight-loss stories with thousands of people. What do I have to be embarrassed about? My scar is a small chapter in a much broader and greater journey. I am not embarrassed about losing half my body weight, completely reforming my life, and creating the healthy life I had always dreamed about.

I beat obesity and came out with a scar. I will take it! I like to think of my scar as a BA battle wound—it's like the ones the heroines have in the movies, the women who have an amazing body and a sexy battle wound that depicts how tough they are and where they've been. While I am not kicking butts and taking names, I did conquer obesity. That was my battle. My tummy-tuck scar is my battle wound. I will never be embarrassed about any struggle I endured on my journey.

More information on loose skin and tummy-tuck recovery can be found in Chapter 8.

How did you actually stay committed? That is my biggest struggle.

It's not easy committing to a goal when you don't make it something you enjoy doing. I was so tired of dreading the gym. I was exhausted with having to convince myself that "diet food" could be yummy.

I wanted to be healthy but I found nothing enjoyable about it. I was stuck trying to convince myself to love all the wrong things. I tried the quick-fix methods. I attempted the fad diets. I forced myself to complete exercises that were just not for me. All of it left me drained and dreading every day of my "healthy life." So I changed things up.

I found workouts that I loved, workouts that made me want to go back. I discovered exercise that left me feeling energized, accomplished, and motivated, not defeated, crushed, and like a fat failure. I fell in love with being vegan. I discovered that peanut butter and toast is an awesome breakfast. There were tons of healthy food options that I had been blind to because I was hyperfocused on how much I hated my "healthy" life. I almost gave up because I was tired of living a life I didn't enjoy for a goal that was slowly becoming out of reach in my head.

So I changed my mind-set. I realized that if I wanted to reach my goals, I would need to stop viewing the end goal as a deadline and more as a way of life. I needed to create the life I wanted to live. I was living a life that I hated and chasing a goal that I was ready to give up on. So I found my passions: Healthy foods. Teaching group fitness classes. Sharing my story. Listening to others' stories.

Working out with my husband and my mom. Breaking a sweat and laughing with others while staring at each other with the "Can we actually complete this workout?" look. I love it! I love everything about my life.

If you feel like giving up, change your game plan. Don't change your goals. You deserve to be healthy and happy.

I do okay during the week but when the weekend comes, I can't control myself and eat all the junk food. What can I do to stop sabotaging my progress?

This is such a common experience. You're not alone. All that planning you put toward your week—meal preparation, scheduled workouts, diligent grocery shopping—is not a Monday through Friday occurrence only. There are seven days in a week. You should be preparing seven days' worth of meals. You will eat food Saturday and Sunday, so that means you must prepare food for Saturday and Sunday. You cannot leave things to chance when it comes to reaching your goals. If you set yourself up for success by preparing your meals for Monday through Friday, why would that change on the weekend?

Prepare your weekend meals. Plan your weekend grocery shopping. Organize your weekends the way you would your weekdays. It's not that you're a failure and unable to practice self-control; more often, you're simply not allowing yourself to be successful. You are not taking the extra steps by prepping food for the weekend, and that is causing you to have problems staying focused.

What if you do prepare your foods for the weekend and you do plan ahead, yet you're still unable to control your eating habits on the weekends? What if no matter how much planning and diligent preparation you practice, you still end up eating way more than you intended, and eating foods that are not going to get you closer to your goals? This could be a result of undereating throughout the week. When your body is starving, or simply not receiving enough calories during the week, when the weekend comes and you're around food more, your body will *want* to eat more. You will find yourself overeating and overindulging because your body is trying desperately to find nutrients and fuel.

So if you're experiencing weekend hang-ups, evaluate if you're either not preparing for the weekends or not eating enough during the week. Both situations will cause the same experience: unplanned overeating on the weekend. Take time to evaluate what the root could be.

My family likes to eat at restaurants a lot, and I find myself not knowing what to order. How do you stay on track when eating at a restaurant?

I like to eat at restaurants too. Healthy eating does not have to mean you must be isolated from all forms of social interaction when food is involved. You can be healthy and interact socially with food involved. It's about being smart and understanding the basics of healthy eating. It's not rocket science. Don't feel like you need to dedicate countless hours to reading nutrition books and exploring the latest studies in the nutrition education world. You do not have to be a walking encyclopedia of nutrition in order to be successful on your journey. What is important is that you understand what healthy eating looks like for you and what foods your body responds best to. What form of healthy eating gives your body the best results? That is what matters.

So when eating at a restaurant, with your individualized healthy eating methods in mind, stick to the basics:

- Vegetables are your friends. Order them. Order lots of them. Search for dishes that are primarily composed of vegetables and start there. Ask how the vegetables are cooked. If they are cooked in butter, ask to hold the butter. Since I don't eat meat, oftentimes if I order a dish and ask to hold the meat, extra vegetables will be added upon request. When I eat at a restaurant, I will always find the dish that offers the most vegetables and see how I can "veganize" it.

- If you're eating at your family's favorite burger restaurant, order the meat alternative patty. They tend to be lower in calories, and veggie patties are delicious. You do not have to be vegan or vegetarian in order to appreciate a good veggie patty. If you can't bring yourself to order a patty made of vegetables because that just doesn't seem "natural" to you . . . that's okay. I won't judge you. Look for lean meat options and avoid the heavily sauced, cheesed, and baconized burger options. You can't reach your goals if your burger sends you into cardiac arrest. I also opt to have my veggie patty wrapped in lettuce rather than served with a bun. The bun is another waste of calories and I prefer the addition of a crisp lettuce wrap.
- Going out to an Italian restaurant? Whole-wheat pasta is your friend. If you haven't noticed, I like to refer to healthy foods as "friends." I think that way because healthy foods treat my body well. I see results when I eat healthfully. Healthy foods are good to my body and helped me reach my goals. Yay for healthy foods! Whole-wheat pasta is your friend and will help you reach your goals.

  Whole-wheat pasta topped with garlic, basil, and roasted vegetables—that's a pretty simple dish and I'm sure an Italian restaurant will have something similar on its menu. Again, make swaps and adjustments when you need to and always ask about the sauce that is used. Oftentimes, heavy cream sauces top otherwise healthy dish options. You can always ask for sauce on the side or pick a different and lighter sauce. While this might sound "picky," keep in mind that all the little steps you take will add up to big changes in the end. By flexing your healthy choice muscles more often, they will grow stronger than your unhealthy habit muscles. What muscles are you going to strengthen? It's your choice.
- Say *no* to cheese. I follow this guideline because I'm vegan. However, cheese is a calorie bomb. Add cheese to restaurant-sized portions and it's more like an atomic calorie bomb. Cheese, while delicious, is something that can add colossal amounts of calories. Oftentimes, people underestimate the caloric value of cheese and

overestimate its serving size. Macaroni and cheese, grilled cheese sandwiches, cheeseburgers, cheese sticks, multi-cheese nachos, cheese bread, cheese pizza with a cheese-stuffed crust, crackers topped with cheese spread and toasted shredded cheese, etc. are all cheese-based favorites that when served with restaurant-sized portions will have you reaching your daily calorie goal with just one meal. When I was vegetarian, cheese was my main food group, so much so that I gained weight. If you're going to continue to consume cheese, do so with a purpose. Practice portion control and pay attention to your daily calorie intake. When eating at a restaurant, I highly encourage you to ditch the cheese and cheese-based meals. Stick to dairy products at home so you can ensure you're eating the right amount and not enough for a small army.

- Salad toppers can be diverse and loaded with nutrients. Or they can be calorie bombs that make your salad as heavy and calorie dense as a fried and cheese-smothered dish. There are two different types of salad topping categories:
  - Salad Topping Category One: diced apples, chopped vegetables, sunflower seeds, slivered almonds, fresh raspberries, blueberries, dried banana chips, black beans, kidney beans, hummus, fresh chopped cilantro, dried or fresh basil, chopped green onions, diced tomatoes, hemp hearts and seeds, sliced hard-boiled eggs, fresh deli cuts, freshly squeezed lemon, vinaigrette dressings, orange segments, etc.
  - Salad Topping Category Two: crispy bacon bits, croutons, crispy onions, crushed tortillas, fried chicken, shredded cheese, diced packaged meats, ranch dressing, creamy blue cheese dressing, candied walnuts or almonds or peanuts, etc.

These two distinct categories of salad toppings will contribute completely differently to your weight. One option will help you lose weight and the other will contribute to weight gain. If you are ordering a salad at a restaurant, watch the toppings that come with it. Avoid the fried and crispy options. Some salads at chain restaurants pack just as many calories and just as much fat and sodium as a giant bacon cheeseburger. Simply calling something a salad does not make it healthy. Having lettuce at the bottom of a bacon, cheese, fried chicken, ranch dressing, crispy onion, and crouton dish does not constitute a salad. If that is what you're eating, why even order a salad?

There is more to a salad than lettuce. Think fresh options, like fresh fruit and chopped vegetables. Get a healthy crunch from nuts, seeds, and diced apples. Enjoy a kick from freshly squeezed lemon and fresh sweet and tart raspberries. Protein can come from beans, fresh sliced lean meats or meat alternatives, or sliced hard-boiled eggs.

Salads can be filling and scrumptious if you want them to be. Gone are the days when salads consisted of wilted wet lettuce, a tomato slice, and shredded carrots. You can make salad exciting and flavorful. See what other options a restaurant has that can be added to your salad. Since I order my meals without meat and cheese, I often ask if I can add some toppings from the other salad options to my salad.

- Avoid fried and crispy options. This equates to calories, fat, sodium, and lots of oil, and it will not bring you closer to your goals. You want to look for the baked, grilled, or steamed options. Baked chicken or tofu, steamed vegetables, grilled fish and meat, these options are much lighter in calories and will help you stay on track.
- Check out the menu online before you leave for the restaurant. In my family, if dinner was going to be eaten at a restaurant, sometime in the afternoon a text would go out to everyone. It would be from either my parents or whoever decided that dinner should be at a restaurant. A few more text exchanges would take place until the group decided on what restaurant to eat at. Once I knew which restaurant, I could go online and check out its menu. I did not have to feel a sense of "Oh no! What am I going to eat? Will they be able to serve me and my special dietary needs? Will I be able to stay on track?!"

  I did not have to stress about dining out because I could access the menu and decide what I was going to order before I even arrived. Checking the menu online also allowed me to search their allergen section so I wouldn't need to rely on the server to find out if the house sauce contained dairy or eggs. Search online before you leave and decide what you're going to order. You will arrive at the restaurant feeling prepared and not stressing over what you're going to eat.

- Don't feel compelled to eat the side that comes with your dish.You don't need to eat the french fries just because they have come with your order. Ask for something else. Check out the side dish options and ask to substitute the fries for a bowl of fruit, a side salad, or some steamed vegetables. Unless the restaurant has the best fries ever, it's not worth it to me. If I'm going to indulge in some french fries, you better believe they need to be either crinkle-cut fries or thick steak-cut fries. I'm not going to waste a treat meal on some wilted and soggy regular fries that don't even look cooked all the way. So if you're at your favorite restaurant, use your planned treat meal. Just don't get into the habit of making every time you eat at a restaurant a time for a treat meal. Treat meals should not be an everyday occurrence. I have always stuck to one or two treats a week. I like to save mine for my date nights with Dre over the weekend.
- Think of making healthy swaps. If the group you're hanging out with is craving ice cream or something cold and sweet, recommend a frozen yogurt shop. With all the various flavor combinations, your group will still be pleased with frozen yogurt over ice cream. Many frozen yogurt shops provide dairy-free fruit-based sorbets that are perfect for those of us watching our calorie intake. For topping options, you can choose to go healthy and add fresh fruits, chopped nuts, granola, and coconut. Your friends can have all the candy bar, chocolate, and cookie and cake crumble options they want. It's the best of both worlds. You get a healthy sweet treat that still keeps you on track, and your friends get their sugar-rush cold-and-creamy fix.

It's my birthday soon, so what can I eat to still stay within my goals?

When it's my birthday, I will eat what I want. I will have healthy foods and I will have unhealthy foods. I will have vegan treats for myself, and

I will have traditional treats for the partygoers. Because not everyone who attends my birthday celebrations eats the same way I do, I like to provide foods that everyone will enjoy, including me. At my birthday parties (typically hosted by my mom), you will find:

- Vegetable and hummus trays including celery sticks, carrots, olives, broccoli, cauliflower, and sliced green and red peppers
- Fresh fruit platters including sliced strawberries, watermelon, blueberries, cantaloupe, sliced pineapple, and sliced apples
- A cracker and cheese tray
- My homemade chocolate and peanut butter no-bake cookies
- A bowl of dark chocolate–covered almonds
- A dish with mixed nuts (I like to add semi-sweet chocolate chips to make a sweet-and-salty snack bowl)
- Build-your-own-sandwich platters including a variety of sliced bread choices (wheat, whole grain, white, rye, etc.), various fresh deli meat slices, toppings (lettuce, pickles, tomato slices, onions), cheese slices, and condiments (mayonnaise, relish, hummus, mustard, etc.)

  The sandwich platter is a great way to allow people to make their own sandwiches however they want while you still get the option to make a healthy sandwich. Again, this way you will be able to host a party that will keep you happy and healthy without "forcing" your guests to be like you.
- Chips (tortilla, pita, barbecue, potato)
- Chips are my favorite and a *must* at my birthday party.
- Dips (hummus, salsa, cream-based dips, etc.)
- Cookies and cake

  These are sometimes vegan and sometimes not, depending on whether or not I decide to bake. I don't always have a cake for my birthday; sometimes I just don't want one. My mom will purchase a regular cake (typically carrot, because that is Dre's preferred cake) and we will serve that.
- Dairy-free ice cream (made from soy milk, almond milk, coconut milk, etc.)

My dad will always buy me some dairy-free ice cream for any event at which cake will be served so I don't feel "left out."

Now out of that list, what things do I personally eat at my birthday party? You will see me with my plate loaded with no-bake cookies, chips and salsa, pita chips and hummus, fruit, and some vegetables with hummus. I will routinely frequent the chocolate-covered almonds bowl and grab handfuls of mixed nuts with chocolate chips. I will most likely make a sandwich with the vegetables options (adding extra pickles) and add some hummus and mustard. I will eat the same things until the party is over, but you will always find me by the chips bowl. My birthday party treats are planned. I am prepared to eat treat food for my birthday party and I thoroughly enjoy myself. I've been known to throw down on chips and salsa! However, I do not keep the leftovers. I do not keep the extra cookies. The extra chips are bagged up and either sent out with guests or stored away (where I won't see them on a regular basis). The vegetable and fruit trays are saved, but everything else that is "tempting" for me—primarily the chips and the chocolate goodies—are sent away or discarded.

Why do I get rid of everything? I find a new place for all the extra food because moderation does not work for me. I will continue to eat the cookies until all the remaining plates of them are gone. I will eat through bags of chips and still want more. While I *can* control myself when unhealthy foods are in my house now, it was not always that way. My journey took five years and I have since been in weight maintenance mode for two years. I've had a while to work on developing some lasting healthy habits.

Before I developed my self-control strength, I would get incredibly frustrated when I heard people say, "Well, just eat in moderation." I couldn't do it. Moderation works for people who've never had a problem to begin with. I had a problem. If food was left available to me in an uncontrolled way, I would abuse it. Moderation was a method that set me up for failure. It drove me crazy time after time, because everyone else seemed to be able to stop eating when they were full. Not me. I always wanted more. I could always eat more than everyone else and then want food again shortly after completing a meal.

It was not until I began to limit my access to such foods that my ability to say no grew stronger. Not everyone will struggle with saying no, and that is great. However, a majority of us on our weight-loss journey do struggle with saying no. It's an almost impossible task and the thought of ever being able to master the ability to turn foods down seems impossible. The simple task of walking into the staff room at work and avoiding the free doughnuts on the table is unbearable. If food is available, you will eat it. Even the foods you don't enjoy too much, if openly available to you, you will eat. That's a scary feeling to struggle with, knowing that you can't turn food down. Every time a peer brings cookies to class you can't help yourself and grab three or four on your way out the door. If candy is on the counter while visiting an office, you take a few pieces. You don't even know how long it's been there and yet you still grab it! Anytime you enter the grocery store you leave with a few cases of cupcakes and a liter of soda.

You engage in that behavior because you have a problem with food, plain and simple. Whether it be an addiction, poor coping skills, lack of stress management abilities, or disordered eating habits, you have a problem with food. That is why your weight is out of control and you're currently at rock bottom. I am here to tell you that it does get easier over time to say no, but you will have to practice daily healthy eating skills and strengthen your healthy habit muscles. I enjoy my birthday party and then the foods are put away. It's a birthday party, not a week-long ordeal.

Other people reading this might be thinking, *What the heck! It's your birthday party! Enjoy the freaking cake and have fun. Stop stressing over your weight and eat some effing cookies!* And that is because everyone will have different struggles. You, my friend, don't have a problem saying no to food, so you don't know the struggle. That is okay! You're not expected to understand something that you don't struggle with. If this is you, then enjoy your cake at your birthday. Just know that not everyone can eat a piece of cake and stop there, so for those people, it's important to have a plan.

More information about developing healthy food habits and applying moderation, as well as other food-related topics, can be found in Chapter 4 and Chapter 7.

As a vegan, or even just as someone who eats healthfully and wants to lose weight, how do you manage family holidays like Thanksgiving and Christmas?

Being vegan doesn't equal having only salads and grass as meal options. Unfortunately, that is a common misconception on what vegans eat. I am routine in my ways of eating. That is how I managed to have a successful weight-loss journey, because of my learned ability to plan ahead and stick to the plan. I eat the same things for breakfast every day, not because I'm boring, but because I enjoy my morning bowl of oatmeal and blueberries. I enjoy toasted English muffins with peanut butter as a mid-morning snack. I could eat the same types of foods every day and be okay. Who would turn down a frozen-cherry and banana smoothie topped with shredded coconut? Not me. So I am 100 percent okay eating my "boring" vegan foods. I find them delicious and they have helped me reach my goals. I fell in love with eating simple food because the results followed.

When Thanksgiving and Christmas arrive, these are opportunities for me to flex my nonexistent vegan culinary muscles. This is the time when I search for yummy holiday-inspired vegan recipes and attempt to make them. I find a balance between healthy dishes and indulgent dishes. It's the holidays, so I want to enjoy the traditional holiday flavors . . . but I don't need to sacrifice my goals for three pieces of pumpkin pie (during Thanksgiving, you know you're guilty of eating more than one slice of pie!). I spend Thanksgiving at my parents' house, where my mom and I work well in the kitchen together. Okay, she basically does the majority of the work and I'm her sous chef. But I always have a few dishes that I *need* in order to feel that my vegan Thanksgiving was a success. I need stuffing, mashed potatoes, rolls, and some kind of dessert. I aim to find a balance between healthy indulgence and holiday indulgence.

That balance looks a little different every year. I am still learning how to handle the holidays, when overeating is the expectation. For the past few years I have focused on creating healthier versions of my favorite dishes. Stuffing can be made on the healthier side. In the past I have added delicious and nutritious ingredients to my stuffing: sautéed onions and mushrooms, sunflower seeds, chopped celery, and low-sodium vegetable broth. I'll use a good stuffing bread mix that meshes with my attempt to keep Thanksgiving on the lighter side. This is a healthier alternative to an otherwise heavily sauced, breaded, and buttered dish. The sweet tooth aspect of Thanksgiving is where I branch out the most. My mom and I discovered a great apple crisp recipe the very first Thanksgiving we tried to keep things on the lighter side. Since that very first healthier Thanksgiving, it's been a holiday regular. I adapted it to make it vegan, so it was still able to grace our family table when I made the switch. It's one of the favorite dishes of my mom and me; I think this is because it holds so many memories.

Our very first Thanksgiving that was focused on healthy eating was shortly after we joined the weight-loss program I talked about in Chapter 1. We were so excited to tackle Thanksgiving with a healthier twist. We adopted the holiday food approach: "Fill your plates with islands, not continents," which is the portion-control idea where you don't pile your food high on your plate. Your food items should not touch each other because you're making islands. We still use that phrase around the holidays to this very day.

Every year Thanksgiving is a little different for me. Some years I have focused more on the healthier side and other years I have indulged more. Ultimately, I still reached my goals. So it will come down to you and your abilities. I do not have a hard time breaking up with Thanksgiving food the following day because it does not include my favorite types of foods (chips and dip are my weakness, and that is not a Thanksgiving food option at my household). I love Thanksgiving, but I am able to move on the next day and not feel compelled to continue to eat the leftovers.

Ultimately, I make my own vegan dishes: stuffing, mashed potatoes, rolls (which are store-bought, because I'm not that good of a cook), mushroom gravy, and no-bake cookies. I accompany my dishes with green salad, sweet potatoes, yams, green beans, and fresh corn. And that is how this vegan does Thanksgiving. I share my stuffing and dishes with those who want to try them. Typically, guests don't even know these dishes are vegan and will keep going back for more. So my dishes are gone by the end of the night, and I feel stuffed and ready for bed by 6:00 p.m. The next day I wake up, everything is back to normal, and I eat my bowl of oatmeal with blueberries.

That's how I do Thanksgiving. Christmas is similar. Add a baked ham or two to the family table, but my approach is the same. I will prepare a few healthy dishes, splurge a bit, and enjoy the day. In my mind, it's one day. It's similar to the birthday question asked and answered earlier. Find what works for you. I make dishes and bring them for myself and to share. If you're celebrating the holidays at another house, bring your healthy options with you to share. Use this as an opportunity to make that recipe that caught your eye a few weeks ago. Have a blend of indulgent options and healthy options and enjoy the night. The following day, eat healthfully, exercise, and enjoy your life. One day of unhealthy eating won't ruin your life the same way one day of healthy eating won't take you to your goals (unless one day of being unhealthy sends you spiraling out of control . . . don't live by that motto; find a motto that supports your goals).

I know some people focus on ratios: For every splurge item eaten, have two servings of something healthy. Or drink a glass of water before you sit down to eat. Or don't go back for seconds until thirty minutes after eating. All of these methods might work for them . . . but I know what works for me is having both options available. I eat for myself, and I enjoy my family. I don't eat enough for fifteen people. I don't eat an entire cake by myself. I share my beloved peanut butter and chocolate no-bake cookies. But most importantly, I enjoy the company around me and have good holiday food.

Remember, you're creating a life to enjoy, not a life filled with restrictions and complicated diets.

More information about developing healthy food habits, moderation, and other food-related topics can be found in Chapter 4 and Chapter 7.

What does a typical week of exercise look like for you? What did exercise look like for you while on your journey?

The first part of the question is more relevant for my weight management years, as people want to know what I am doing right now to keep my body in the shape it is in. I don't share the specific breakdown of my exercise routines (i.e., I do X number of repetitions of this workout, run X number of miles, and use X amount of weight when I do squats, etc.). This is for three reasons:

- I might currently be completing an in-home workout program that can be purchased. In that case, I share the name of the program with the person asking so they can look into purchasing it.
- My current workout schedule is packed with classes that I was or am teaching and/or attending. In that case, I will share the name of the format and encourage people to find a local class in their area.
- I could currently be completing an individualized or coached plan designed for my own personal goals, in which case it would irresponsible to share this plan with someone for whom it is not specifically designed.

Regarding what my exercise looked like while on my journey, this question is hard to answer because my exercise style has changed so dramatically over the last five years, or even the last seven years if you include the time I've been maintaining a healthy weight range. What I do now is completely different from what I did when I first started. What I did while in the middle of my journey is completely different from what I did toward the end of my journey. Your exercise routines will vary depending on what place you are currently at in your journey. When I first started my journey, I hated exercise. I hated the gym. I hated gym clothes. I actually didn't own any gym clothes when I first started my journey. I wore sweats that doubled as pajama bottoms and old church camp T-shirts. My first serious experience with exercise was at an all-female gym I joined with my mom. It had a circuit-style-training setup, where you'd use a machine for a specific interval time and then move off and hop onto the next machine, and so on. I went through the motions. I put absolutely zero effort into my "workout." I hated it. I loved going with my mom. I loved the people who worked there. I loved the people who exercised there. I just could not find any sense of enjoyment from that type of exercise.

My mom and I would attend at least five nights a week. Eventually, that dropped down to my only going two nights a week until I stopped altogether. I tried to find ways to make myself enjoy it more, but I just couldn't. My mom and I joined the "advanced" circuit, so the intensity was stepped up. I was sure that would bring me results! But I still had to put forth the work . . . and I wasn't willing to.

When that phase ended for me, I found myself signing up for a personal trainer at my local gym. My mom stumbled across a bikini-body challenge the gym was promoting and thought it would be "good" for us to sign up. I agreed and signed up. I hated it. I hated the workouts. I *really* hated the gym. I hated the mirrors, and the incredibly fit people made me feel bad about myself. I hope you are sensing the trend of my terrible attitude at this point in my journey. I had a bad attitude about anything fitness related. I hadn't found anything that made me *want* to work out . . . so I walked around with animosity toward fitness and was spiteful toward all the fit-looking people. I wanted to look like them . . . but I was unable and unwilling to put in the work.

My personal training experience lasted eight weeks. In that time I dropped a few pounds but my workouts diminished from the recommend six days a week. I was lucky if I managed to get in two workouts a week. A few weeks after my personal training experience ended, my mom and I stumbled across a Zumba presentation at our local fair. It looked like so much fun! I love to dance, and I wanted to lose weight. So I figured, why not try something that combined both?

My mom and I attended our first class the following week. *Boom!* I was hit with the fitness bug. I had finally found something that made me *want* to work out. I looked forward to attending classes. We started attending classes six days a week, sometimes two classes a day. I was not a morning person, but I would wake up early on a Saturday to attend the morning Zumba class. Zumba made me fall in love with exercise. Fitness clicked for me at that moment. I was doing everything wrong up until that point in my journey. I needed to find something that I enjoyed, something that made exercise not only bearable, but fun. For me, that was Zumba.

Exercising became a weekly routine at that point. I would attend classes five to six times a week. I went off to college and continued to attend not only Zumba but also other classes as well, such as cycling, boot camp, strength classes, etc. I branched out into a whole new world of group fitness classes because I fell in love with one form of exercise. That passion and excitement I felt from Zumba made me want to find more exercises that made me feel that way.

Fast-forward one year, and I began teaching Zumba classes myself. I added additional personal workouts from the in-home program I received as a Christmas gift, the one that had me crying on the floor because it was so intense. I was teaching four classes a week (Zumba and cycling) and then I added the in-home program, which consisted of six workouts a week. That's a lot of exercise! My body embraced it. I was challenging myself in a way I never had before and my body was drastically changing as a result. I followed the meal guide that came with the program and my weight just began to fall off. I was eating the right things, eating enough, eating responsibly, and busting my butt . . . and the results followed. I went from a size twelve/fourteen to a size six in sixty days.

I was now hooked on fitness. I craved it. I loved my daily workouts. All it took for me to get that fitness bug was to find something worth getting excited about. Once that excitement was there, everything else became so much easier. I didn't dread the gym. I had days when I got dressed a little slower, but I no longer sulked and pouted the entire time. I put forth effort in my workouts. I paid attention to my intensity and heart rate. I *cared* about what I was doing. I desired to improve my fitness abilities. I was on my way to looking like those fitness girls I envied at the gym back when I was just starting my journey.

Since that point, my workout schedule has remained pretty similar: five to six days a week, with one dedicated rest day. My workouts themselves have varied tremendously. I joined a strength training gym and attended group classes that combined strength training with cardio bursts. I completed other in-home workout programs that incorporated athletic and sports endurance training methods. I even dropped the cardio and dedicated myself to an intense, concentrated strength training program while I trained for a bikini competition.

My exercise has varied depending on where I was in my journey; it varied dramatically between weight-loss mode and weight maintenance mode, and it also varied based on what goal I was currently trying to reach. What remained the same was my five- to six-day dedication to crushing my workout with high intensity and focus, and moving my body with a purpose. Find *your* fitness style and you will release your inner fitness god/goddess.

More information on my fitness journey can be found in Chapter 3, Chapter 5, and Chapter 6.

What are your next fitness goals? What are you striving for now that you're done losing weight?

It's always a strange experience when I stop to remember that I have actually reached the top. I made the switch to weight maintenance . . . and it seemed to happen overnight. One day I was striving to lose weight and the next day I was done reaching that goal. It's been two years and it still throws me off when I stop to think about it. I busted my butt for five years, so it's not unusual that it's taken some time to adjust to maintaining weight versus losing weight.

A focus on creating fitness goals has helped make the transition easier. Establishing fitness goals gave me a sense of purpose, as odd as that sounds. Regaining my health was my purpose for so long, and I did it. I completely transformed my life, my body, and my outlook on life, and I reached the top of Mt. Weight Loss. Yay! I found good health. But then what? I was left feeling goal-less. I felt a lack of purpose. My workouts felt stagnant. What was I going to do now? The past five years of my life had been focused on one central goal, and I had reached it. So what would come next?

I realized that I was ready to take on more challenges and create new goals for my well-being and body. Weight loss is one narrow facet of the broader domain of health. I could check off the weight as an area of concern in my life and focus on something new. The positive thing is that I was healthy and am healthy now. I no longer have to worry about weight-related illnesses, or dread going to the doctor's office because my weight will be talked about. I actually dreamed about what it would be like to walk into the office of the doctor who told me that I would never be small, that I just "wasn't built that way." I wanted to see the look on his face when I stepped on the scale and he looked down at my chart to see the weight change.

That never happened, though. He was at my family doctor's clinic for only a short time. However, when I came in for a routine checkup with my new family doctor, who had not seen me in four years, she had to double-check her chart to make sure she was seeing the right patient. That made me feel good. That almost made up for not being able to see the male doctor—almost.

I did it. I reached my goal . . . And now it was fitness time. I set various new goals for myself; some have been met and some are still a work in progress:

- Be able to do a pull-up unassisted (work in progress)
- Get visible abs (completed)
- Run a long distance without stopping (completed: seven miles without stopping)
- Improve my sprinting speed (work in progress)
- Complete the advanced versions of my favorite in-home workout programs (completed: earned the T-shirts to prove it)
- Be able to climb a rope (work in progress)
- Train for and compete in a bikini competition (completed: two times)
- Run a marathon (work in progress)
- Complete an obstacle run (work in progress)
- Improve my flexibility through yoga (work in progress)

- Obtain my personal training certification (work in progress)
- Be able to do a proper-form single-arm push-up (work in progress)
- Expand my group fitness résumé (completed: I have taught and can teach cycling, strength, conditioning, boot camp, Zumba, and MixxedFit classes)

My "Work in Progress" list is long, so I've got plenty of things to keep me busy, focused, and ready to kick butt at the gym. I will always be a goal digger.

I don't like water. How can I make myself learn to like it?

Water was hard for me to learn to drink too. I struggled for a long time! I actually did not begin drinking plain water until *after* I reached my goal weight. All of a sudden my stomach could no longer handle the sugar-free flavor packets I was adding to my water bottles. My stomach would become painfully bloated, to the point where I would cringe in pain whenever I moved. I reached out to a friend who is a practicing holistic food counselor. She shared with me that my water habits had to change. I wanted to live in denial, because plain water was just not for me. But I also just couldn't bring myself to keep engaging in a habit that was causing me so much pain. I was also experiencing debilitating headaches. I was a mess. I stopped adding the flavor packets to my water, and my body went back to normal. No more bloating. No more painful headaches.

I did not drink plain water on my journey, I added flavor packets to my water, and I still reached my goals. I cannot tell you to avoid adding flavor packets to your water because of the sugar-free chemicals when I drank them during my entire journey—religiously. I would not have stopped using the flavor packets had my body not freaked out. This will be a personal preference for you. What does a healthy life look like for you? Is it important for you to drink plain water? Is that a goal you have for yourself? Are you experiencing bloating? Could the sugar-free chemicals be a contributing factor?

If you want to begin to learn to drink plain water, set up a ratio system. For every flavored water you drink, you need to drink the same amount of plain water. If you have a goal to drink plain water, start with ratio drinking and then slowly increase the plain water to flavored water ratio (i.e., for every one flavored water you drink, drink two plain waters, etc.). Another approach is to begin reducing the amount of flavoring you add. Add half the packet and then slowly reduce the amount. I've also seen people infuse their water with fresh fruit. "Infuse" sounds fancy, but essentially you are simply adding fresh fruit slices to water. It's nothing crazy, but it can provide a hint of fruity sweetness and flavor to the water.

I can't attest to the sugar-free chemicals found in water flavoring hindering weight loss, because I drank them. All the time. Dre and I drank flavored water all the time. Brea and I drank flavored water all the time. We would purchase massive amounts, in all different flavors, and drink them endlessly. I did not drink plain water, ever (except when I was teaching fitness classes).

This will be an area of personal preference. I can't argue either way. On the one hand, I lost over one hundred pounds while drinking flavored water. On the other hand, they eventually gave me debilitating headaches and massive digestive issues. It's up to you to decide if you want to add them to your water.

If water flavoring is not your thing and you simply want to learn to drink more water in general, purchase a nice water bottle and carry it everywhere you go. If you're into technology, you can purchase "smart" water bottles that will track your water intake for you and alert you when you need to drink some. Even I would benefit from something reminding me throughout the day to drink more water. I carry around a water bottle with me everywhere I go and that helps me drink water. It also keeps my hands busy so I don't feel tempted to reach for goodies I encounter throughout my day. Plain water is still a new thing for me. When I was in college and graduate school, if I was drinking liquid it was either espresso or flavored water. Coffee is your blood type when you're in graduate school!

I feel like I'm never doing enough. If I am not sore the next day, I assume the workout I completed was wasted. After a workout I always wonder if I could have pushed harder and done more repetitions. How do I know if I'm actually working hard enough?

You're pushing yourself incredibly hard during a workout. Your arms are shaking, you're covered in sweat, the floor beneath you looks like a puddle, your lungs are burning, and your heart is pumping. Your workout ends and after five or six minutes you feel fine. Your heart rate is normal. Sweat has dried up. Now you're looking at yourself in the gym mirror wondering why your body is not still in pain because only a few minutes ago you thought you were going to pass out.

You're a rare breed. You're a fitness extremist. You crave the endorphin rush fit for Olympian athletes. You're also too hard on yourself. When your body shows signs of exhaustion, it's not pretending. Your body is not trying to trick you into thinking that you're working harder than you actually are. You *are* working hard, but you're in shape. Your body recovers quickly because you've conditioned your heart and your muscles. That does not mean that your workout was wasted and that you didn't accomplish anything. You will not be sore after every workout. Not every workout will be a marathon sprint. You will not feel incapable of walking after every single leg day. That does not mean you did not work hard! Do not get into the habit of measuring your workout effectiveness by how sore you are the next day. While it can be "fun" (which is a relative term) to be unbearably sore, because it makes you believe that you kicked some serious butt during your last workout, equating soreness to workout effectiveness is also a dangerous mentality.

It's dangerous because your body will not always be sore after a workout, which will lead you to continue to increase the duration and frequency of your workouts That will jeopardize your body's ability to heal and repair after a workout. What used to be a forty-five-minute high-intensity workout will turn into a sixty-minute high-intensity workout. This will then lead to sixty minutes of high intensity followed by thirty minutes of concentrated strength training. You will continue to add segments and additional time to your workouts until you eventually overtrain and cause yourself a serious injury.

To know if you're "actually" working hard enough, invest in a heart rate monitor. Monitoring my heart rate was one of the greatest training techniques I ever introduced into my workouts. A heart rate monitor allowed me to track how hard I was really working, not just how hard I thought I was working. I could see what heart rate zone I was reaching. I was able to track how quickly I recovered. I was able to learn my resting heart rate. I could see my max heart rate and know when I was pushing myself to the best of my ability. If you are not sure if you're working hard enough, invest in a heart rate monitor. It tells you the calories you've burned and some other information, but most importantly, you can track your workout intensity. You will be able to definitively know if you are maxing yourself out. So there will be no more questions and no more doubts.

Do not let yourself fall victim to thinking that you're not working hard enough. Don't allow your desire to reach your goals make you push your body beyond your abilities. You do not want to cause an injury that could have been avoided had you stayed within your abilities and trained smarter. Athletes do not train at the risk of hurting their bodies. If you want to look like an athlete or a fitness model, train like one. Athletes pay attention to what their bodies are telling them. Monitor your intensity, but don't measure your workout effectiveness by how sore you are the next day. Take care of your body, be diligent with your workouts, and stay within your abilities.

I'm worried that after I lose weight no one will love me because of loose skin and stretch marks. I'm so embarrassed about what I will have done to my body, I could never let someone see me naked.

Stretch marks and loose skin are not unlovable traits. You are not less of a person because you once were or currently are overweight. Being overweight is not the worst thing a person can be. I understand the daily struggle of feeling that your weight is completely and utterly out of your control. I know how it is to feel like the entire world is looking down on you because of how much space you take up. I understand that you sense the disgusted looks everywhere you go. I get it. I've been there. But I am telling you that you don't have to stay in that negative mental space. You can choose to be happy. You deserve to be happy. God did not put you on this earth so you could spend your entire life hating yourself.

You can find someone who loves you for you, but first *you* have to love you. I don't think the issue is fear of not finding someone who will love you. What I see is that you're worried no one can love you because you can't even love yourself. There is a reason I started the very first chapter of this book with the topic of self-love. Self-love is the driving force for this journey. Self-love will be the reason you get up and keep moving after you get knocked down. You must love yourself enough to work harder. You must love yourself enough to know that you deserve to live a healthy life you're proud of, not a life full of self-hate, doubt, and loneliness.

When you can love yourself, you won't worry about other people's love for you. Eventually, you will find that special someone whom you want to spend the rest of your life with. But for right now, focus on learning to love yourself. Pray. Keep a diary. Keep a journal. Write love letters to yourself. Write encouraging messages to yourself throughout the day. You are your own best friend. You will be the only person who can get you to your goals. You will be the only person who can get you to the top of Mt. Weight Loss, and if you can't even be on your own team . . . how do you expect to succeed?

You need to be your number-one supporter. There will be times on your journey when other people will doubt you. Their doubts can bring you down if you don't have a strong enough will to keep pushing. Focus on your health. Focus on your goals. You have so much to gain by completing this journey. What are loose skin and stretch marks when compared to a lasting life of health, a new outlook on life, and self-love? You have so much positivity to gain when you embark on this journey, and all you have to lose is weight.

Try not to focus on what you can't control. You can't control stretch marks. You can't control loose skin. You can't control when you find the love of your life. You can't control the hypothetical outcome of taking your clothes off in front of someone at some point in your life. You have zero control over all these "what-if" moments. What can you control? Your attitude. Your dedication to your goals. The amount of planning you put toward your meals. The effort you put toward your goals. The way you talk to yourself. The words you use to describe yourself. You have control over these areas. Focus on them! If you're worried, write about it. What are you worried about? Journal your fears and worries, but don't let things end with them controlling you.

You can reach your goals. You will reach your goals. You will learn self-love, so start by practicing it. Start by reading the letter every day that I asked you to write in the introduction. Right now your journey is not about finding romantic love, or worrying about "what-if" hypothetical scenarios. Your journey is about finding self-love. Start there. You cannot reach your goals if you are not on your own team.

I would not be the person I am today without 256-pound Sharee busting her butt. I will never be embarrassed about where I have been, because I wouldn't be here without my past experiences.

More information on self-love, loose skin, and stretch marks can be found in the introduction and Chapter 8.

I still have no idea how to decide how I want to eat while on my journey. Where do I even start? There is so much information out there! How do I know what will work for me?!

Getting started is overwhelming. There is so much information out there. Just when you think you've found something you might enjoy, in, for example, the exact same magazine you're reading, you will find an article conflicting with what you just read. Even nutritionists disagree over what is healthy and unhealthy. How can you navigate through a world where even the experts and certified specialists can't agree on anything? With so much information out there, you have to take a step back, take a deep breath, and focus on your goals.

When you think about a healthy person, what do you see? What is your idea of a healthy life? When envisioning your ideal healthy person or the person you aspire to be like, what do you like about their approach? When thinking about the person who inspires you and what their methods and approach were, keep in mind that just because a specific diet worked for them does not mean that it will be right for you. However, what can be discovered from exploring how your inspirational figures eat are your ideas and a place to start. At this point in your journey, you don't know what will work best for you and your body. You don't know if your body will respond to a low-carb diet, veganism, simple clean eating, etc. You can't compare these new dietary choices to each other because you are starting at ground zero.

The pro? You can pick any way of healthy eating and see if your body will respond well. Pick one way of eating and try it out for a few weeks and see how you feel. Are you seeing results? Do you feel energized and vibrant? Or do you feel tired and sluggish? It's overwhelming when you see all the different ways of eating, but just focus on one and try it out. You have nothing to compare it to because you're just starting out. Keep in mind that you can't "fail" when trying out different ways of eating; you simply will learn what works well for your body and what doesn't.

Low carb is not something my body responds well to. Even prior to becoming vegan, I tried a low-carb diet because that is how my dad likes to eat. I was not successful. I have come to learn that my body has a natural aversion to low carb. I like my carbs! These are things that you will learn too. Keep a food journal and track not only your intake but also how you're feeling. Do you feel healthy—not the Sarah kind of "healthy," where you associate starvation with being healthy—but are you actually feeling energized, refreshed, and happy?

Now you won't feel happy all the time, and eventually you will be offered some foods you'll need to turn down. But you can feel happy the majority of the time because you're taking positive action for your health. While this process of getting started can be overwhelming, remind yourself daily that this whole experience is a learning process and that it takes time. You're also not expected to hit the trails sprinting and know everything there is to know about healthy eating. You're just getting started. Allow yourself time to learn what this process will look like for you. Try different things out. Know the basics: whole grains, low-fat dairy options, lean meats or meat alternatives, healthy fats, fruits, and vegetables are better for you than processed, refined, and packaged foods. Take those staples of healthy eating and find what ratios and varieties of the foods will work for you. If you begin to feel overwhelmed again, remind yourself that you are learning what will work for you. That process will take time. Don't panic and don't freak out. You will find what works best for you. I recommend taking some time to complete the "Getting Started" guide found in Chapter 12.

More information about eating habits, healthy foods, and different eating styles can be found in Chapter 4 and Chapter 7.

Are all the fancy gadgets—microchip running shoes, step trackers, heart rate monitors, fitness trackers—worth it?

I will share what I used on my journey. I had the popular training shoes that came with the microchip. The microchip was located in the bottom of the left shoe and it tracked my pace, distance, calories burned, stride length, and other similar running stats. The microchip sent all the information to my phone and/or my computer. I was able to see and hear all my stats while I ran.

I purchased these shoes with the intent to increase my desire to run. It didn't work. I used them for a few weeks. I tried to learn to like running. The information I could track was really useful and cool to have acess to. That was the first time I began to have goals of one-mile running times. I wanted to run faster and farther. But the excitement quickly faded for me; I just don't enjoy running.

If you enjoy running or want to try to get into running, the shoes might be useful for you. It was motivating to see my stats and running details. Some online programs have coaching modules that sync with the shoes. This allows you to create a plan to help you increase your distance and speed, or even train for a race like a marathon, a half marathon, a 10k, etc. If you want to try running, the shoes can be a fun present to give yourself, or something to ask for around the holidays or your birthday.

I've used both heart rate monitors and fitness trackers. What is the difference between the two? A heart rate monitor tracks your heart rate, calories burned, duration of exercise, max heart rate reached while exercising, and average heart rate during exercise. Heart rate monitors are worn only during exercise. Most options have a chest strap you put on right before you begin to exercise. The strap has the sensors that measure your heart rate and the data is displayed on the wrist piece. Some heart rate monitors and dual-functioning fitness trackers will have heart rate sensors built into the wristband.

A fitness tracker records the steps taken per day, provides you with a daily step goal, calculates calories burned throughout the day, and monitors sleep patterns. Some will monitor your heart rate all day and others will monitor your heart rate only during exercise. A fitness tracker has more options in terms of what it records compared to a heart rate monitor that is primarily used just while exercising.

I purchased a heart rate monitor while on my journey and it helped me understand my intensity levels. I was able to see and gauge the effort I was putting toward my workouts. The scale does not always reflect how hard you're working. If I became frustrated with the scale, I was able to refocus my mind-set and remain positive because I *knew* that I was putting forth the effort in my workouts. My body was just having a weird day or an off week. But I was bringing my A-game to my workouts.

I feel that technology can make your workouts enjoyable and can give you feedback that you don't get from the scale. The scale can't measure improvements in your resting heart rate. The scale can't show how you're able to recover faster between intervals. A heart rate monitor or fitness tracker can help you set new fitness goals. The scale can't show you that you walked ten thousand steps yesterday as opposed to your average three thousand. A fitness tracker will help you pay attention to movement that you would otherwise never think twice about. How many steps on average do you get in a day? When you have a daily step goal, you will find yourself moving more, parking farther away, and taking the stairs. When you're aware of your movement, or lack of movement, you will begin to change your behaviors.

I personally enjoy both of them. I like tracking my daily steps. I like knowing my resting heart rate. I pay attention to my heart rate while working out. I love knowing the total calories I burned at the end of a workout. Fitness trackers help hold me accountable to my goals. To me, they are a positive investment. If you want a way to hold yourself accountable to reach daily fitness goals, and to ensure you're exercising with intensity and purpose, I suggest you consider adding a fitness tracker or heart rate monitor to your routine.

What was your tummy-tuck recovery like?

It was no walk in the park, I will tell you that right now. But it was worth it. If for some reason I ever had to have another, I would do it again. I had an amazing doctor and nursing staff who walked me through every step of the process before I had my surgery. They did not sugarcoat the recovery. I did not walk in the day of surgery and have unrealistic expectations about the recovery process. I knew it would be long. I knew that parts of my recovery would be painful. I knew I would struggle mentally and emotionally. They prepared me, the best they could, to be able to face all of it.

When I was just waking up from the surgery, I had to go to the bathroom urgently. I was still groggy from the anesthesia, so my movements were sluggish and I tried to sit up while on the surgery table. The nursing staff told me to move slowly and lie back down. I looked at them and said, "It's okay, I work out." After a few minutes I was taken out to my mom's car in a wheelchair and sent on my way home. My surgery was six and a half hours long. I showed up at 6:30 a.m. and left the office around 2:00 p.m. I slept the majority of the car ride home. My body felt really stiff. I didn't have any pain, I just felt stiff. When I got home my mom and Dre helped me sit in a recliner chair and that is where I slept for the next two weeks.

When I woke up the day after surgery, that's when the pain set in. I had drain tubes on both sides of my lower stomach . . . That was gross. The drain tubes helped the excessive fluid leave the body (super gross). The swelling hit me like a ton of bricks the second day. I was huge, bruised, bloody, and still trying to figure out my pain medication dosage. My body had a negative reaction to the pain medication, which gave me a panic attack. In the middle of the night I tried to take off my compression suit and demanded that my mom search me for extra incisions. The medication was making me hallucinate; I felt like I was crawling out of my skin, and I couldn't stop crying. After my mom reduced my pain medication dosage, I felt normal and comfortable.

Once my medication dosage was sorted out, the recovery process was smoother. Again, I slept in the recliner chair for two weeks. My abdominal muscles were so tight, they felt as if they would rip in half if I were to stretch out too much. I developed a hunch when I walked, so I had to mentally remind myself to stand up straight. I was able to comfortably stand up straight around day fifteen. The actual pain itself was not immense. I was sore, stiff, tired, and bruised, and I felt like I had just undergone major surgery. But I did not feel tears-streaming-down-my-face pain. Except when I sneezed . . . Which was awful. Don't sneeze after a tummy tuck.

I underwent my surgery during finals week and spring break. After seventeen days of recovery I went back to class. I was no longer on pain medication because I needed to drive and function. There was also no way I could function in a graduate-level statistics course while under the influence of heavy pain medication. So I used generic pain medication and iced my body regularly. Adjusting to school life after major surgery caused many emotional breakdowns. I was physically and mentally exhausted after completing even the simplest tasks. Sitting in a desk all day caused my swelling to increase, and that in turn caused me to be irritable and get agitated. A trip to the grocery store was something that I could celebrate because all I wanted to do was sleep. Recovering from major surgery is incredibly strenuous on the body.

The hardest part of recovery is not the physical aspect or the pain. The hardest part to overcome is the mental aspect. You go from being in the best shape of your life, which in my case meant teaching group fitness classes five-plus times a week and completing personal workouts, to not even being allowed to lift five pounds. The smallest tasks exhausted me. But although the recovery was slow, I always knew that it would be worth it.

After eight weeks I was cleared to resume workouts. There are no restrictions on workouts, so of course I wanted to go back to my super-intense, killer workouts . . . But I was unable to complete even one push-up. My abdominal muscles were essentially brand-new and had never been trained, strengthened, or conditioned. Although my arms and legs remained strong, my core strength was gone. You don't know how much core strength goes into various exercises until you no longer have a strong core! I was frustrated. I had anxiously waited for weeks to be cleared to work out, and now my workouts would have to be modified.

I was too embarrassed to attend any group fitness classes, not because of my surgery but because I did not know what fitness abilities my new body would have. I knew what my old body could do. My old body could easily complete rounds and rounds of push-ups, teach classes back to back, and do burpees for hours. With my new body, I was not sure what I could do. I did not want to be in the middle of class when I found out that I couldn't complete a sit-up or a side plank. I just wanted more time to learn where my new body was fitness-wise. I started with light cardio on a stationary bike and then progressed from there.

I incorporated two to three workouts a week. If I tried to add any more exercise, my swelling increased to painful amounts. I was still icing my body and wearing my compression suit every night. The swelling was taking its time to decrease, but it was decreasing. They don't call it "swell hell" for nothing. As the days and weeks passed, I began to feel better about myself. Initially, because of the swelling, none of my clothes fit. I could wear only stretch pants and baggy shirts. Eventually, the swelling began to decrease and I was able to ease into wearing some of my old clothes. Then one day, I wore my very first crop top and jean shorts out to the store.

I stared at myself in the mirror in disbelief. I used to be 256 pounds, and now I was able to walk around in a crop top and tiny shorts. I was so proud of myself. I asked Brea to take pictures of me before we left the house so I could share the moment on social media. I began teaching fitness classes about four and a half months post-operation and my life began to feel "normal" again. I still struggled with core strength for the first eight to nine months. I even experienced some random pain when I attempted to climb a rope twelve months post-operation. My body took time to adjust, but I did start to feel normal again, and now there is nothing I can't do.

I married the love of my life six months after my tummy tuck and our honeymoon in Mexico was the first time I ever wore a bikini on the beach. A tummy tuck is not an easy procedure to endure, but in my opinion, it's not the most painful.

If you're considering getting a tummy tuck, research your doctor beforehand and look at the "before" and "after" pictures on the surgeon's website. Find a picture of someone with loose skin similar to yours and see if you like their results. What I noticed and liked the most about my surgeon's pictures were the belly buttons he had created. You do not get a new belly button when you have a tummy tuck, but the incision for your belly button is new. It is in the same spot and has the same internal structure; it's just a new outside hole. Sometimes the belly buttons surgeons have created look odd and misshapen; they turn out looking unnatural and botched. My surgeon created a great belly button hole for me, which turned out really cute.

I also paid close attention to the scar and incision-line placement. Some surgeons place scars higher than others. While this will also depend on how your loose skin falls on your body, I knew I wanted a low scar. That is something I discussed with my surgeon during our consultation, how low he could make my scar. Research your doctor and find someone who can answer all your questions and make you feel comfortable about the process. You will have many post-operation visits, so you want to make sure you enjoy the staff and your doctor.

I worked so hard this week and when I weighed myself, I had gained five pounds! How is that possible? Now I feel like giving up.

Welcome to the sick, twisted games hosted by the scale. I hate that feeling. I hate when I know that I worked freaking hard all week and the scale decides to show a two-pound increase. The scale is a lying cow, I'm just going to throw that out there right now. The scale does not measure your effort, dedication to your goals, healthy food habits, or the times you worked out even though you didn't want to. The scale measures the relationship between your body and earth as determined by gravity. Weight gain is not fat gain. Just because you gained weight does not mean you gained fat. There are thirty-five hundred calories in one pound. In order to gain two pounds, you would have to consume seven thousand extra calories in addition to the calories you burn from being alive. You did not gain two pounds of fat. Weight gain on the scale can be a reflection of water retention, sore muscles (sore muscles retain water), sodium (high or increased levels of sodium can cause water retention), hormone imbalances (i.e., menstrual cycle), etc. There are lots of reasons the scale will show an increase despite how hard you worked that week. That is one of the reasons I have opted to weigh myself once every two weeks versus once a week.

When I was on my journey I would get so discouraged when the scale did not reflect how hard I thought I had worked that week. When I began to weigh myself less often, I did not see the fluctuations caused by water retention. Eventually, I went to weighing myself once a month. Now in weight maintenance mode, I don't pay attention to the scale unless I am training for something. Or I might step on the scale to check that I am still on track, for my own mental peace of mind.

I used the scale on my journey to ensure I was moving in the right direction and eventually began to look at other ways to measure my progress, such as clothing size, how my clothes fit, how I felt, muscle definition, and body measurements. The scale measures one area of your journey, but it does not measure the whole journey. It cannot show you all the progress you've made. That is why it's so important to have other goals and measurement methods to track your progress. The scale will not tell you if your mile time has improved. The scale will not show how much lean muscle mass you've built. The scale won't tell you how many inches you've lost off your waist. The scale can't tell you how much more weight you can bench-press. The scale won't show you how much you've improved in your Zumba class.

The scale does not measure your entire journey. It measures your weight. There is more to this journey than losing weight. Focus on all those areas. Weight is only one area. What about your food habits? Have they improved? Are you making healthier food choices? Are you snacking on apple slices when you used to eat chips all the time? Has your water intake increased?

What about your fitness? Can you run faster? Can you jump higher? Can you complete more challenging exercises? Do you find yourself attempting new forms of exercise? Has your strength increased? Is your endurance higher? There is so much more to this journey than what the scale can show you.

I always feel bad when I have a treat meal. How can I make that feeling go away? I want to be able to enjoy my treats and not feel bad.

Think of healthy eating like homework scoring. Let's say you eat three meals a day (I eat about five meals a day, but for this example, we'll go with three). Three meals a day seven days a week equals twenty-one meals per week. That means that throughout the week, you have twenty-one opportunities to make healthy choices. Monday and Tuesday you stick to the basics and eat your favorite healthy foods. Wednesday arrives and you go out to lunch with your co-workers to your favorite bakery. You have your beloved toasted sandwich with chips, and finish the meal with the bakery's signature double-chocolate-chunk muffin. Thursday and Friday there are no surprises with your foods. You worked most of the day and brought all your meals from home. Saturday you attend a movie with a friend and order a large popcorn with your favorite candy. On Sunday you meet your family for brunch and order the French toast topped with vanilla ice cream and strawberry slices.

You ate twenty-one meals and three of them were treat meals. That means that eighteen of the meals you ate that week were healthy. Eighteen is 85 percent of twenty-one. So you ate healthfully 85 percent of the week. Since when is an 85 percent bad? Eighteen out of twenty-one is a great ratio. What you do every day matters more than what you do every once in a while.

If you feel yourself worrying about every treat meal you have, think about your week. Was this a good week? Did you stick to your healthy meals? What's this week's score? One or two treats a week is not going to set you back, unless those treats last a whole day and then leak into the weekend. It's hard to not feel guilty, but please focus on the positives, not the negatives.

If you find yourself continually feeling guilty anytime you eat a treat meal, track your "food homework." See what your healthy meal to treat meal ratio is. It can help ease your mind and remind you that your everyday behaviors shape you, not the every-once-in-a-while behaviors. It will take some adjusting to not feel guilty every time you stray from your typical foods. But don't let guilt control you. This is your healthy life, not your guilty life. If anytime you eat a cookie you second-guess your food choices, that is not a fun life to live. This is a life you *want* to live. You want to enjoy your life and there is nothing enjoyable about feeling guilty. Find that balance. You can have cookies while on your journey. Just be smart about it. Understand what works for you. If you need to take a break from cookies, take a break (i.e., moderation is not an option for you right now). Enjoy your treat meals and enjoy your healthy meals. Find what will work for you and your body. Find the method that your body responds well to. Some people have one treat a day and other people have one to two a week. I prefer one to two treats a week; my body responds well to that. Other people have treat days . . . that wouldn't work for me. A whole day of treats would make it easier to have treats the following day, and so on. I really enjoy my treats!

Find what works for you. This entire process is a learning experience. There will be bumps, but that's life. This is your journey to create a healthy, happy, amazing *you*. That will take time, so enjoy some cookies along the way. Just make sure to embrace those healthy foods too.

Besides losing the weight, what was the hardest thing you had to overcome on your journey?

A big challenge was understanding that losing weight takes time and that it takes work. I felt that since I wanted to lose weight . . . it should just happen. I thought that by going through the weight-loss-method motions the weight would just fall off. Weight loss does not work that way. Body transformations are not made by simply going through the motions. I had developed this sense of entitlement toward weight loss. I felt entitled to it because I was so burdened by my weight. I felt that mentally accepting it was time to lose weight would be enough to initiate the weight-loss process. It's almost like I thought that since I had been overweight for so long, I had endured enough and done my "part." I had zero work ethic in relation to weight loss and transforming my life.

This was not because being healthy was a foreign concept to me; both my parents were healthy. I just *wanted* to be skinny but did not want to put in the work that it takes to be skinny, thin, and healthy.

I remember sitting in nutrition classes during one of my first quarters of college. These were the annoying classes that everyone was required to take for an undergrad degree, but that don't actually apply to a bachelor's degree. Fast-forward five years, and I would love to take a nutrition class now. But back then, not so much. I attended the class every day, but I never paid much attention. I already "knew" all the information. I knew what healthy eating looked like. I knew that is was important to exercise. I knew that saturated fats should be avoided. But there I was, two hundred and some odd pounds, and I thought I knew everything about losing weight. I just didn't want to do the work and accept responsibility for my actions. I would say I matured the most when I moved to Scotland and had a wake-up call with food, when I was forced to not only "know" what healthy eating is but also practice it. What a concept.

Eventually, my work ethic grew and branched into fitness as well. When I matured in both areas, my weight loss dramatically increased. That was over a span of three years and it was a tough learning process for me. I had to learn that you actually have to engage in the behaviors and take the actions that will get you to your goals. You can't just talk about engaging in them, or think about doing them . . . you have to actually follow through. Mind-blowing, right? If I wanted to look fit, I had to do what fit people do: exercise. If I wanted to be healthy, I had to do what healthy people do: not eat junk food.

I'm not the only one who struggled and still struggles with this concept. Someone reading this right now might have just had an enlightening moment, a realization that you can't just want something, study it, read about it, and pretend to do it. You have to actually dedicate yourself to it, practice it, embrace it, and give it your all. You won't reach the top of Mt. Weight Loss making only a 75 percent effort. It doesn't work that way. You need to give this journey your all. One hundred percent makes up a successful weight-loss journey. Ninety percent is an "I almost made it" story. Don't be an "I almost made it" story. When I learned, the hard way, that I needed to give 100 percent, I pouted for a bit and then got serious. You can't lollygag around and expect to lose a hundred pounds. Either you want to get in the best shape of your life, lose weight, and reach your goals, or you don't. There is no middle ground. You can't halfway want a goal. Commit to your goals and create a plan to get you there.

I lost only two pounds this week. I worked really hard and just feel so discouraged because this process seems to be taking forever. I hate how long it takes to lose weight.

Life is not microwavable. There is no quick-start button. There is no "land on this space and you get to move ahead four spaces," because life is not a board game. With education and career development, you can't take a shortcut to skill mastery. Weight loss is the same way. There are no shortcuts. There are different methods, and some work more effectively than others, but there are no shortcuts that result in lasting healthy weight loss. There are no quick fixes. This process takes time. The sooner you accept that, the easier the process will become. Weight loss is hard. Creating a fit body is hard. Reforming unhealthy eating habits is hard. But is hard a bad thing?

When did hard become something that must be avoided? You don't develop when things are easy. When people share their life-changing moments, the moments that shaped their skills and molded them into who they are today, they don't talk about walks on the beach or a warm and cozy coffee date. Their personal accounts are gut-wrenching stories about overcoming hardship and giving everything they had to reach their goal: that difficult moment defined. The only way you can grow is when you're challenged. You will not change, grow, and develop if you're comfortable.

Hard is not bad. Embrace hard work. This process will take time. You will have to work hard, and keep working hard, for an extended amount of time. That is okay! You will grow. You will develop lasting skills to help you maintain your weight loss. Hard work might not be the preferred method, but it's the only option that will get you to your goals and keep you there. Weight loss will not be a one-way trip unless you take the time to develop the skills to keep you at your target destination. Weight loss can become a round-trip, really quickly.

You're bummed you lost only two pounds? How would you feel if that was two pounds gained? Would two pounds still be a small number then? It's doubtful. You would flip out. You'd question your methods. Wonder if you're working hard enough. Worry that you're not eating the right things. Scrutinize every single food choice you made that entire week. If the scale is moving in the right direction, stop questioning the process. I know you want to drop twenty-five pounds in a few weeks, but that much weight loss is unrealistic and incredibly unhealthy in such a short amount of time. Weight loss will take time! Allow the process to work. Save all the questioning and evaluating for if the scale begins to significantly move the other way. I started my journey twice. The second time I decided I was no longer going to look back. And I didn't care how long it took. Taking any number of steps in the right direction is itself a step in the right direction. Don't get hung up on the amount of time it will take to reach your goals. Just decide that from here on out, you will start to make a conscious effort to reach your goals.

This guy or girl broke my heart and I'm trying so hard to not turn to food for comfort right now. What can I do to keep my mind off food and this crappy situation?

I've been there. Breakups suck. Heartbreak is hard to get over. Turning to food might seem like a good idea right now, but think about the bigger picture. This is an opportunity to use an appropriate coping strategy. It's a sucky situation, but still a good learning opportunity and a chance to work on replacing unhealthy eating habits with healthy habits. So what can you do instead?

- Talk to a friend
- Call your mom or dad or siblings
- Write out a long rant and send it to your friends
- Work on a puzzle
- Download a new game on your phone
- Go for a walk or jog or sprint
- Lift some heavy things at the gym
- Paint or draw a picture
- Color in a coloring book
- Go to a coffee shop and start writing
- Read your favorite book or magazine
- Get a manicure
- Invite a friend over for your own mani/pedi time
- Go shopping for a cute dress or shirt or shoes or rings, etc.
- Get all dolled up and take cute selfies
- Go outside and smash things with a hammer (in a controlled setting)

- Go to a pet store and cuddle with puppies and kittens (or cuddle your own pets)
- Rip up old phone books

These are some ideas of activities that can help you handle your emotions without turning to food. A lack of coping skills can lead to overeating. Focus on engaging in activities that will help you cope with the situation, not run from it.

Final Thoughts

If I had to look back over my entire journey from start to finish, I would say the very beginning of it was that moment when I cried in the car with my mom—the moment after seeing 256 pounds on the scale for the very first time. I sat and cried, overwhelmed by a sense of self-sabotage, defeat, and frustration. The end of my journey would be when I wore a bikini on the beach in Mexico while on my honeymoon . . . five years later. I walked across the beach and felt amazing. I felt healthy, strong, fit, and happy. I had just married the man of my dreams and I looked like the girl whom I grew up daydreaming about.

I went from a girl crying in the car and feeling so hopeless about her weight, so lacking in control over food and her life, so overwhelmed with the burden of needing to lose one hundred pounds . . . to a girl who is passionate about health, fitness, and self-love. I went from hating how I lived my life to loving everything about my life. Over those five years I completely and utterly transformed every aspect of my life, to make it the life I had always wanted. Throughout my journey, I cried, prayed, screamed, yelled, sweat, bled, and contemplated giving up. But I stuck with it. You can too. Stay strong; this journey is nothing you can't handle with the right plan in place. When you feel motivated, plan. When you feel overcome, burdened, and alone, pray. When you feel like giving up, remember why you started. I will never go back to being the girl who cried in the car with her mom. Fight for your health. Take charge of your habits. Enjoy the journey and celebrate your accomplishments along the way. Remember, it does not matter how long it takes you, as long as you're moving in the right direction.